The Speech-Language Pathologist
From Novice to Expert

D1314961

Arthur M. Guilford
University of South Florida

Sandra V. Graham
University of South Florida

Jane Scheuerle
University of South Florida

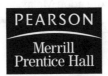

PEARSON

Merrill
Prentice Hall

Upper Saddle River, New Jersey
Columbus, Ohio

Library of Congress Cataloging-in-Publication Data

Guilford, Arthur M.

   The speech-language pathologist: from novice to expert / Arthur M. Guilford,
Sandra V. Graham, Jane Scheuerle.

      p. cm.

   Includes bibliographical references and index.

   ISBN 0-13-153463-7

   1. Speech therapists—Study and teaching. 2. Speech therapy—Practice. I. Graham,
Sandra V. II. Scheuerle, Jane. III. Title.

   RC428.5.G853 2007

   616.85′50071—dc22

                                                2006016178

Vice President and Executive Publisher: Jeffery W. Johnston
Acquisitions Editor: Allyson P. Sharp
Editorial Assistant: Kathleen S. Burk
Production Editor: Sheryl Glicker Langner
Design Coordinator: Diane C. Lorenzo
Production Coordination: Karen Ettinger, Techbooks
Cover Designer: Jeff Vanik
Cover Image: Super Stock
Production Manager: Laura Messerly
Director of Marketing: David Gesell
Marketing Manager: Autumn Purdy
Marketing Coordinator: Brian Mounts

This book was set in Palatino Roman by Techbooks. It was printed and bound by
Bind-Rite. The cover was printed by The Lehigh Press, Inc.

Pearson Prentice Hall™ is a trademark of Pearson Education, Inc.
Pearson® is a registered trademark of Pearson plc
Prentice Hall® is a registered trademark of Pearson Education, Inc.
Merrill® is a registered trademark of Pearson Education, Inc.

Pearson Education Ltd.   Pearson Education Australia Pty. Limited
Pearson Education Singapore Pte. Ltd.   Pearson Education North Asia Ltd.
Pearson Education Canada, Ltd.   Pearson Educación de Mexico, S.A. de C.V.
Pearson Education—Japan   Pearson Education Malaysia Pte. Ltd.

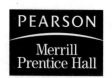

10 9 8 7 6 5 4 3 2 1
ISBN: 0-13-153463-7

This book is dedicated to all those mentors and colleagues who have contributed to our own personal and professional development and to our students whose achievement of expertise in speech-language-pathology we may have influenced.

Preface

One of the greatest rewards of being a speech-language pathologist is having the chance to give back to the profession. Our discipline, like those of other helping professions, has benefited from the efforts of many individuals in different settings who have contributed through teaching and mentoring students; who serve on boards and committees that oversee legislation and policies, programs of study, and service providers; who conduct and publish research; and who carry out the day-to-day practice of the profession. Ours is not a "self-study" type of discipline. The entire professional community contributes to the development of new speech-language pathologists and fosters their continued professional development.

We have dedicated ourselves to developing our own levels and areas of expertise. It is our hope that through this book's content, students will develop an understanding of the profession's requirements for practice and an attitude that will enable each to embark on a journey toward professional fulfillment and expertise.

This book presents and discusses various aspects of when and how speech-language pathologists develop expertise. Learning objectives focus on understanding the features of expertise, how speech-language pathologists pursue expertise, and characteristics of practice settings in which expertise may develop. The book's content targets undergraduate and graduate students in the beginning stages of professional preparation. Practicing speech-language pathologists too may find this material a refreshing review and update of practice in varied settings. The text considers historical perspectives of expertise and ways in which speech-language pathology has drawn from other professions. Issues integral to development of expertise receive consideration, such as cultural diversity, professional standards and conduct, and evidence-based practice.

Part I provides an overview of the concept of expertise in several disciplines within the helping professions. It addresses particular implications for the concept of expertise as it relates to the speech-language pathology profession. A model provides a framework of expertise in speech-language pathology and component clusters (we call them factors) of the model's features.

Part II discusses each of the model's components as it relates to current professional issues and trends. This section provides opportunities for self-evaluation and for the reader to formulate a personal plan for professional development from novice to expert.

Part III examines expertise in many speech-language pathology practice settings, including schools, hospitals, private practices, nursing homes, rehabilitation facilities, and university programs. Experts from each of these areas share knowledge and experiences specific to the type of setting and provide guidance for developing expertise.

The book supports both beginning and practicing clinicians with a comprehensive look at how their developmental continuum from novice to experienced professional to expert might unfold in the various settings where speech-language pathologists practice and progress toward expertise. Following a summary, each chapter offers a series of thoughts for exploration. These thoughts encourage introspection and application of the chapter's information. Although this book points out major mile markers along the journey to professional expertise, much of the journey is unique to the individual clinician. This book provides information that assists clinicians in formulating their own plans for the professional growth and development that lead to expertise.

ACKNOWLEDGMENTS

We appreciate the hard work of all the contributing authors. They are: Tempii Champion, Ph.D., Department of Communication Sciences and Disorders, University of South Florida; Jacqueline J. Hinckley, Ph.D., Department of Communication Sciences and Disorders, University of South Florida; Nancy J. Huffman, CCC-A/SLP, Consultant, Churchville, NY; Alex Johnson, Ph.D., Department of Audiology and Speech-Language Pathology, Wayne State University; Peter Johnson, Ph.D., Speech Mentor, Select Medical Rehabilitation Services; Linda Rosa Lugo, Ph.D., Communicative Disorders, University of Central Florida; Russell Malone, Ph.D., American Speech-Language-Hearing Association, Retired Communications Director; Michael Moran, Ph.D., Communication Disorders, Auburn University; Arlene Pietranton, Ph.D., American Speech-Language-Hearing Association, Executive Director of ASHA; Fred Spahr, Ph.D., American Speech-Language-Hearing Association, Retired former Executive Director of ASHA; Nancy Swigert, M.A., Swigert & Associates, Inc., Lexington, KY; and Kathleen Whitmire, Ph.D., American Speech-Language-Hearing Association, Director ASHA School Programs.

We would like to thank the reviewers who provided invaluable comments and suggestions. They are: Kathryn Adam, Rush University; Linda C. Badon, University of Louisiana at Lafayette; Julie Fuller-Bolling, Eastern Kentucky University; Monica Devers, St. Cloud State University; Carol Myhre, Minnesota State University; Laura M. Piche, State University of New York (SUNY) Geneseo; Sara Elizabeth Runyan, James Madison University; Dale Williams, Florida Atlantic University; and Brenda Wilson, Eastern Illinois University.

Discover the Merrill Education Resources for Communication Disorders Website

*T*echnology is a constantly growing and changing aspect of our field that is creating a need for new content and resources. To address this emerging need, Merrill Education has developed an online learning environment for students, teachers, and professors alike to complement our products—the *Merrill Education Resources for Communication Disorders* Website. This content-rich website provides additional resources specific to this book's topic and will help you—professors, classroom teachers, and students—augment your teaching, learning, and professional development.

Our goal with this initiative is to build on and enhance what our products already offer. For this reason, the content for our user-friendly website is organized by topic and provides teachers, professors, and students with a variety of meaningful resources all in one location. With this website, we bring together the best of what Merrill has to offer: text resources, video clips, web links, tutorials, and a wide variety of information on topics of interest to general and special educators alike. Rich content, applications, and competencies further enhance the learning process.

The *Merrill Education Resources for Communication Disorders* Website includes:

- Video clips specific to each topic, with questions to help you evaluate the content and make crucial theory-to-practice connections.
- Thought-provoking critical analysis questions that students can answer and turn in for evaluation or that can serve as basis for class discussions and lectures.
- Access to a wide variety of resources related to classroom strategies and methods, including lesson planning and classroom management.
- Information on all the most current relevant topics related to special and general education, including CEC and Praxis™ standards, IEPs, portfolios, and professional development.
- Extensive web resources and overviews on each topic addressed on the website.
- A search feature to help access specific information quickly.

To take advantage of these and other resources, please visit the *Merrill Education Resources for Communication Disorders* Website at

http://www.prenhall.com/guilford

Contents

Part II   The How of Becoming an Expert   41

Chapter 5   Developing Interpersonal Skills   43

Chapter 6   Developing Professional Skills with Membership in Professional Associations   52

Chapter 11   Speech-Language Pathology Services in the Schools   118

Chapter 12   Speech-Language Pathology in Nursing Homes, Rehabilitation Facilities, and Community-Based Service Providers   132

The What and Why of Expertise

INTRODUCTION

Part I gives a broad description of expertise and explores the ways in which experts have become acknowledged and valued throughout the human services professions. As one of the modern human-services disciplines, speech-language pathology has a responsibility to its consumers, as to itself, to identify and describe the characteristics of expertise in clinical practice. In the discipline of speech-language pathology, one finds various levels of knowledge and skills among clinical practitioners. Through reflection and assessment, those differing levels of ability can be arranged on a continuum from novice to expert.

In Search of Expertise

Expertise   The conscious and purposeful employment of specialized knowledge and skills in order to achieve exemplary outcomes.

INTRODUCTION

The speech-language pathology profession has gained the respect and regard of other health-care professions and maintains many complex interdisciplinary relationships by continually seeking to provide its best professional services to individuals and groups with communication disorders. In the process, clinical practitioners frequently glimpse expert performance in themselves and in their colleagues. On a larger scale, the speech-language pathology profession continues to seek explanations, definitions, guidelines, and directives that can assist each clinician's progress from novice to expert.

Social issues and trends have significant impact on industry, commerce, education, and health-care services. Demands for efficacy, fiscal accountability, and access help shape professions in these times. Another important trend is consumer education. Health-care consumers must educate themselves to stay abreast of approved scientific advances and to advocate for themselves. These societal movements send consumers in search of the best services and the best professionals for their health-care dollars. Their search for excellence challenges professions and professionals to meet their expectations. In professional circles, the "best professional" is referred to as an expert. This leads us to ask the questions:

- What makes an individual an expert?
- Who is considered an expert in the profession of speech-language pathology?
- How did these professionals achieve the distinction of expert?

Commitment to ethical conduct and to delivering quality services are traditional characteristics of members of all helping professions. This level of commitment, along with a conscious sense of responsibility, drives professionals to be "the best" for their clients/patients and for their chosen profession, as well as for themselves and their professional reputations. This determination is particularly evident among professionals in helping professions. **Helping professions** include medical and nursing care, therapy services, and social and rehabilitative services. Each professional group strives for excellence and expertise. Their members adhere to specific **codes of ethics** and **professional creeds** that identify desired characteristics, roles, and practice parameters. These support professional behavior and aid in decision making. The expert uses these to stay current in all aspects of professional practice. In addition to the influence of codes and creeds, social and professional issues shape the practice of helping professions.

THE INFLUENCE OF EDUCATION AND HEALTH-CARE REFORM INITIATIVES

In recent decades, the helping professions have increasingly responded to demands of consumers, legislation, and funding/reimbursement agencies. As a result, federal legislation such as Public Law 94-142, Public Law 99-457, Public Law 101-476 (IDEA), the 2004 reauthorization of IDEA, and No Child Left Behind (http://www.ed.gov/nclb/landing.jhtml) have helped ensure identification and access to appropriate exceptional education services offered by qualified professionals. Chapters 2 and 11 provide more in-depth discussion of the impact of education reform. Health-care reform has also had a significant impact on the speech-language pathology profession. This impact has influenced the way we deliver services in various settings and influenced the types of clients/patients seen (eligible for services), the degree of services provided (number and length of sessions, setting), and funding for services (preauthorization and funding limits). These initiatives have also influenced the way educational programs teach and train preprofessionals (courses, clinical experiences, methods of instruction, and educational environment/setting). Increasingly complex issues can affect patients, clients, caregivers, preprofessionals, service providers, administrators, and payers. In addition, costs, outcomes, productivity requirements, malpractice, caps on reimbursement, and litigation influence the research and practice of speech-language pathology.

THE INFLUENCE OF DEMANDS FOR ACCOUNTABILITY

As in all human services disciplines, an essential clinical issue in speech-language pathology is caring for client/patient needs in accordance with the **scope of practice.** This is true regardless of the setting or patient/client characteristics. Essentially, this means focusing on treatment efficacy and outcomes. The 1993 establishment of the American Speech-Language-Hearing Association (ASHA) Task Force on Treatment Outcomes and Cost Effectiveness and the 2003 technical report *Evidence-Based Practice in Communication Disorders* demonstrated the commitment of professionals in the field to respond to issues of accountability and quality assurance.

Clinical efficacy is an applied treatment's ability to produce a predicted result. **Clinical outcomes** involve study of the results of either specific treatment methods or general services and the extent to which they are beneficial under typical (real-world) conditions. Efficacy and outcomes vary in their respective degrees of control of conditions and the resulting ability to draw conclusions about cause and effect.

The issues of efficacy and outcomes have been studied from three major perspectives. First, a significant body of research addresses the effectiveness (efficacy) of specific therapy methods. Second, body of research focuses on the identification of functional results of treatment (outcome measures). Third, studies focusing on patient satisfaction contribute to our knowledge base in both areas of efficacy and outcomes (Olswang, 1990). Thus far, research in these areas has focused on the development of treatment protocols according to disorder or handicapping condition, client/patient profiles related to functional outcome levels, and client/patient satisfaction surveys.

Each area of research rests on the premise that the professional demonstrates a set of basic competencies. However, little research addresses the influence of clinician competence levels on outcomes. Although specific competencies may be identified, *degrees* of competence are less easily defined. Each of these factors affects overall treatment outcome. It is important to determine degrees of difference in the individual clinician's professional development or level of competence and the impact on outcomes.

THE INFLUENCE OF EVIDENCE-BASED PRACTICE

Evidence-based practice reflects recent advancements in quantifying efficacy research. This approach, evident in the medical literature since the mid-1990s, has more recently received attention in speech-language pathology practice (Yorkston et al., 2001).

> Evidence-based practice (EBP) is a perspective on clinical decision making that has been described as a paradigm shift in medicine. The EBP orientation, now apparent in fields as diverse as education, pharmacology, and mental health, has the potential to improve significantly the evidence base supporting clinical practice in speech-language pathology, but information about EBP is not yet readily accessible to members of ASHA (ASHA, 2003, p. 1).

We provide a thorough discussion of evidence-based practice in Chapter 7. Several websites provide additional information on EBP. Two excellent sites for EBP in medicine are at http://www.cebm.utoronto.ca and http://www.cebm.net. Two additional sites of value to clinicians interested in searching for evidence concerning conditions applied to EBP are at http://ahcpr.gov and http://guideline.gov.

Service delivery has evolved to the point that customary/habitual approaches to intervention can no longer be accepted without proof (evidence) of the anticipated outcome. Nor can professional decisions regarding treatment (goals, hierarchy for intervention, procedures, techniques, materials, and instrumentation) rely entirely on assumptions and clinical judgment. This is often a major distinction between novice and expert performance. Skilled professionals approach service delivery issues from an empirical basis and provide evidence-based therapy. **Evidence-based practice** has been defined as "the conscientious, explicit, and judicious use of current best evidence in making decisions about the care of individual patients . . . [by] integrating individual clinical expertise with the best available external clinical evidence from systematic research" (Sackett, Rosenberg, Gray, Haynes, & Richardson, 1996). Simply stated, we can consider the basic formula for evidence-based practice as appropriate treatment protocol supported by EBP data + client/patient profile + clinician variables = outcome. The art of the profession (how the practitioner provides the help) is an important but abstract factor. Merging science and art yields a more effective practice.

ASHA has published policy statements related to the designation of competencies associated with the various needs (disorders or conditions) of persons being served. Each **policy statement,** derived from the ASHA Code of Ethics (ASHA, 2003), details the scope of practice, the necessary education and training, precautions, and knowledge and skills needed in the particular area of service delivery. An underlying principle of these policy statements is that identifying the knowledge and skills needed to perform a specific service leads to improved quality of services. Standards of the Joint Commission on Accreditation of Healthcare Organizations (JCAHO, 1988) define **competence** as an individual's capacity equal to the requirements of the position held and views competence as a component of professional qualification. ASHA and JCAHO, however, describe their competencies as performance expectations, not intended to be prescriptive. Each service provider is responsible for defining practitioners' qualifications, including competence, to meet the unique needs of each client in each setting.

THE ROLE OF EXPERTISE

Clinical research has focused primarily on the technical and procedural aspects of treatment. As a result, little empirical evidence identifies, describes, or explains the role of expertise within speech-language pathology. Most of the literature that defines and describes expertise has been drawn from the fields of clinical psychology, medicine, and education (Chi, Feltovich, & Glasser 1981; Chi, Glasser, & Rees, 1982; Clinton, McCormick, & Besteman, 1994; Ericsson, Krampe, & Tesch-Romer, 1993; Hibbard, 1995; Jennings, 1996).

Ericsson and Smith (1991) described studies of experts in selected endeavors (e.g., chess, physics, music, ballet, and figure skating) as attempts to understand and account for the features—described as inherited or acquired stable characteristics—that distinguish outstanding individuals in a specified field from others in the same occupation and from people in general. They concluded that the characteristics that differentiated experts from their colleagues are acquired rather than inherited, are occupation specific, and take a long time to acquire. Additionally, Ericsson et al. (1993) provided evidence to support the proposition that, given innate ability, sufficient deliberate practice, training, and feedback on performance, experts show few limitations to developing expertise. Jacobs (2003) suggests that training can help individuals achieve a certain level of competence, but the individual must make the effort over time to achieve higher levels of development. This is good news for preprofessionals or practicing speech-language pathologists with professional development plans and willingness to commit the time and effort needed to complete them.

Expertise has been described as *what* experts *know* and *can do*. Thus, **experts** are those most capable in specified areas of human endeavor; only individuals who possess the highest levels of competence are recognized as experts (Jacobs, 2003). Identifying an individual as an expert is relatively arbitrary because the levels of ability occur along a hypothesized continuum of competence (Salthouse, 1991). Within selected professions, "expertise" denotes exceptional or extreme performance at the upper end of a normal distribution. Expertise has been found dependent on detailed knowledge of the designated discipline, problem-solving abilities, specialized memory abilities, and inference patterns.

O'Sullivan and Doutis (1994) identified twelve characteristics shared by experts across disciplines. These characteristics, summarized in Table 1.1, are considered distinguishing features of a recognized expert. They include traits, abilities, methods of developing expertise, and descriptions of performance.

The idea of expertise within the speech-language pathology profession reaches beyond the professional's knowledge of communication sciences and disorders. Kierkegaard (1962), Rogers (1958, 1961), Carkuff and Berenson (1967), Cornett and Chabon (1988), Kamhi (1994), Graham (1998), and others suggested that expertise includes not only the intellectual factor, but also intrapersonal, interpersonal, and attitudinal factors. These factors influence clinical decision making, clinician-client interaction, and ultimately, treatment outcomes. The potential benefits of expertise to professional effectiveness make its development important. Developing expertise requires identifying and describing important skills and behaviors. Such efforts also affect clinical practice efficacy and outcomes across the field of speech-language pathology.

TABLE 1.1 Characteristics Shared by Experts Across Disciplines

1. Experts perform complex tasks in their domain much more accurately than do novices.
2. Experts solve problems with greater ease.
3. Expertise develops from knowledge initially acquired by weak methods, such as means analysis.
4. Expertise is based on automatic response to conditions.
5. Experts have superior memory for information related to their occupations.
6. Experts are better than others at perceiving patterns among task-related cues.
7. Expert problem solvers search forward from given information rather than backward from goals.
8. One's degree of expertise increases steadily with practice.
9. Learning requires specific goals and feedback.
10. Expertise is highly occupation specific.
11. Once defined, teaching rules of expertise results in development of experts.
12. An expert's performances can be predicted accurately from knowledge of the rules he or she claims to use.

Knowledge of expertise specific to speech-language pathology is necessary for both practice and research. The study of clinicians and clinician characteristics may reveal aspects and elements of practice that affect treatment and, as a result, relate to the body of efficacy and outcomes research. Specific knowledge about effects of clinical practice and **indicators of expertise** on treatment outcomes is essential to implementing diagnostic and therapy protocols and to predicting treatment outcomes. The clinician may increase the reliability of prognostic estimates of outcomes and increase accountability by combining the following:

- Specialized knowledge of the discipline
- Skill of clinical practice
- Thorough understanding of the efficacy of treatment procedures (National Outcomes Measurement System [NOMS], 2003).

Practitioners, too, benefit from identifying and understanding the characteristics that indicate expertise and how they operate in and influence effective clinical practice. To move toward expertise, the novice must apply considerable attention and energy to the "how" of speech-language pathology as well as to the "what" of diagnosis and treatment procedures and techniques. Each student/novice clinician must discover his or her strengths and weaknesses, analyze each, and modify the weaknesses while increasing the strengths. As he or she learns the strategies and technologies of speech-language pathology, the individual practitioner develops insight into interpersonal interactions, clinical practice, and outcomes. Practitioners regularly interact with peers, teachers, supervisors, clients, and caregivers. Traditional academic activities that target the accumulation of information are enhanced by including opportunities for developing self-knowledge, self-evaluation, rapid recognition of situations for applying knowledge and skills, as well as the relationship of each to clinical outcomes. The beginning professional must become aware of the relationship between level of competence and clinical outcome for the client/patient.

EXPERTISE DEFINED

Expertise is reflected in one's ability to be a confident, knowledgeable, and involved communicator; an integrative thinker and problem solver who simultaneously and effectively quantifies outcomes of treatment, while maintaining the flexibility to adjust to new situations. In addition, the expert clinician in speech-language pathology needs heightened awareness of the scope and limits of his or her interpersonal skills and acceptance of client diversity. In sum, it is no small feat to become an expert in speech-language pathology.

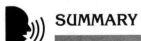 ## SUMMARY

Research has documented the efficacy of specific treatment procedures and the acquisition of anticipated outcomes depending on setting and client variables, and has acknowledged the value of expertise. Although research has identified effective treatment methods, the role of expertise in the outcome of treatment has not been fully established. Prescribed therapy methods and protocols alone cannot accommodate all client and setting variables. We need to continue to define expertise in clinical practice and its role in the intervention process. Knowledge of the novice–expert continuum is beneficial to generate a plan for professional growth and development. Also, the relationship between expertise and treatment outcomes needs to be established, analyzed, and understood.

THOUGHTS FOR EXPLORATION

1. What current trends have influenced client/patient expectations regarding treatment outcomes?
2. How do experts differ from fellow professionals?
3. What effect might level of competence (for example, novice or expert) have on the clinical practice of a speech-language pathologist?

REFERENCES

American Speech-Language-Hearing Association. (2003). Code of ethics (revised). *ASHA Supplement, 23,* 13–15.

American Speech-Language-Hearing Association. (2003, November). Evidence-based practice in communication disorders (Tech. Rep. Draft). Rockville, MD.

Carkuff, R., & Berenson, B. (1967). *Beyond counseling and therapy.* Toronto: Holt, Rinehart, and Winston.

Chi, M. T. H., Feltovich, G., & Glasser, R. (1981). Categorization and representation of physics problems by experts and novices. *Cognitive Science, 5,* 121–152.

Chi, M. T. H., Glasser, R., & Rees, E. (1982). Expertise in problem solving. In R. Sternberg (Ed.), *Advances in the psychology of human intelligence.* Hillsdale, NJ: Lawrence Erlbaum.

Clinton, J. J., McCormick, K., & Besteman, J. (1994). Enhancing clinical practice: The role of practice guidelines. *American Psychology, 49*(1), 30–33.

Cornett, B. S., & Chabon, S. S. (1988). *The clinical practice of speech-language pathology.* Columbus, OH: Merrill.

Ericsson, K. A., Krampe, R. T., & Tesch-Romer, C. (1993). The role of deliberate practice in the acquisition of expert performance. *Psychological Review, 100,* 363–406.

Ericsson, K. A., & Smith, J. (Eds.). (1991). *Toward a general theory of expertise.* Cambridge, MA: Cambridge University Press.

Graham, S. V. (1998). Quality treatment indicators: A model for clinical expertise in speech-language pathology (Doctoral dissertation, University of South Florida, 1998).

Hibbard, S. (1995). *Two studies in expertise and clinical psychodiagnosis.* Knoxville: University of Tennessee.

Jacobs, R. L. (2003). *Structured on-the-job training: Unleashing employee expertise in the workplace.* San Francisco: Berrett-Koehler.

Jennings, L. (1996). *Personal characteristics of master therapists.* Morris: University of Minnesota.

Joint Commission on Accreditation of Healthcare Organizations. (1988). *Accreditation Manual for Hospitals.*

Kamhi, A. G. (1994). Toward a theory of clinical expertise in speech-language pathology. *Language, Speech and Hearing Services in the Schools, 25*(2), 115–188.

Kierkegaard, S. (1962). *The point of view of my work as an author: A report to history.* New York: Harper Torchbooks.

National Outcomes Measurement System. (May 13, 2003). *ASHA Leader.*

Olswang, B. (1990). Treatment efficacy research: A path to quality assurance. *ASHA Leader, 32*(10), 45–47.

O'Sullivan, M., & Doutis, P. (1994). Research on expertise: Guideposts for expertise and teacher education in physical education. *QUEST, 46,* 176–185.

Rogers, C. R. (1958). The characteristics of a helping relationship. *Personnel and Guidance Journal, 37,* 6–16.

Rogers, C. R. (1961). *On becoming a person.* Boston: Houghton Mifflin.

Sackett, D. L., Rosenberg, W. M., Gray, J. A., Haynes, R. B., & Richardson, W. S. (1996). Evidence-based medicine: What it is and what it isn't. Article based on an editorial from the *British Medical Journal, 312,* 71–72.

Salthouse, T. A. (1991). Expertise as the circumvention of human processing limitations. In K. A. Ericsson & J. Smith (Eds.), *Toward a general theory of expertise* (pp. 286–300). Cambridge, MA: Cambridge University Press.

Yorkston, K. M., Spencer, K., Duffy, J., Beukelman, D. R., Golper, L. A., Miller, R., et al. (2001). Evidenced-based medicine and practice guidelines: Application to the field of speech-language pathology. *Journal of Medical Speech-Language Pathology, 4,* 243–256.

Evolution of Speech-Language Pathology as a Human Services Profession

Human Services Professions Professions unique and purposeful in their mission of providing specialized professional services that assist consumers. Human services providers must acquire specialized education and training in order to develop skills and expertise.

INTRODUCTION

Speech-language pathology's widely recognized professional status in current society rests on the creative, untiring devotion of clinicians, researchers, organizers, and advocates and their constant focus on services for persons with communication disorders. The discipline's current philosophy and principles of conduct reflect society and its changes over time.

As a relatively young profession, speech-language pathology has used the collective wisdom of its members to identify and address individuals' communicative needs. Experts have emerged across the scope of practice as speech-language pathologists become recognized leaders in their areas of specialization.

The human services professions are typically those perceived as helpful by the individual who has sought assistance (Richard & Emener, 2003). We tend to see these professions as providing "unique, useful, and purposeful activities by a specialized professional designed to assist consumers with their personalized issues" (p. 8). These professionals provide clearly defined services that require specialized education and training to acquire the expertise necessary to function fully in these professions (Crouch, 1997; Egan, 2002; Emener & Darrow, 1991; Perry, 1996). Careers in human services professions frequently require certification or licensure. Most human services professions require an advanced degree, advanced educational and training standards as agreed on by some governing body or agency, and participation in continued professional development activities to enhance and enrich one's performance. Professionals in these careers should make clearly defined progress toward the mastery of excellence. Advancement toward expertise is not a simple linear progression, however it does develop over time.

A HISTORICAL PERSPECTIVE

Interpersonal communication of ideas and intentions has long been cited as critical evidence of human behavior. Likewise, history notes that a person's apparent failure to develop spoken language has been variously labeled as a shame, a curse, a sign of insanity, and a spectrum of other dehumanizing terms. Through the evolution of diagnosis and treatment of communication disorders, expertise has developed from the culmination of interest, effort, talent, and skill. This type of expertise must respond to societal demands that require and support such services. Likewise, the knowledge, content, and practice within speech-language pathology have drawn on other emerging fields of scholarship and application of theory. That is, the profession that serves individuals with communication disorders could flourish only in a society that reflects the philosophy espoused by John Stuart Mill in 1859, that every individual has the right to pursue the ability to function fully within his or her parameters of potential, age, and place (Mill, 1975). Modern expertise that helps to minimize a communication disorder's effects on the life of the individual, his or her family, and associates can be traced through the evolution of humane responses to the needs of others.

Certainly in earliest eras of human evolution adequate and timely communication were essential for individual survival. Since then, as speech and language have become codified and written, various methods of communication have become more precise and less transient. However, we still need both the ability and opportunity to communicate adequately within our given social milieu. The wide range of communication disorders prevents any single practitioner from becoming expert in every aspect of the discipline. On the other hand, every clinician represents a model of interactive communication and in that role demonstrates skills and traits that attract and sustain the client. As we will discuss in Chapter 3, the foundation for becoming an expert in the discipline focuses on the clinician as a person because the clinician is the basic instrument of change in the clinical process. In other words, the clinician is the most important tool of therapy. This is a common principle of helping professions.

The helping professions embrace numerous disciplines. A feature they have in common is recognition as a profession. The preamble of the American Personnel and Guidance Association's *Ethical Standards Handbook* (1965) identifies three criteria for an occupation to be called a profession:

> The occupation is identified by specialized knowledge, skills, and attitudes. Individuals and society receive services based on a philosophy and code of ethics that earn the provider public recognition and the public's confidence. Practicing members of the occupation have acquired specialized knowledge, skills, and attitudes through prescribed preparation at a college or university, and thereafter through continual updating in professional education.

It is clear that most human services incorporate these criteria and certainly use them as a pathway for progressive professional development from novice to expert.

HUMAN SERVICES PROFESSIONS

Human services professions grew out of observations and interest in the many differences in human health and conditions and from the efforts of a few to diminish the pain of others. Such efforts are recognized among the outcomes of the industrial revolution, the rise of a strong middle class, and increased literacy among the common population. Biomedical investigations through the ages culminated in 19th century assertions about the intimate relationship between neurology, human thought, and behavior (Cole,

1982). These significant breakthroughs led to recognition and valuation of behavioral studies as separate and distinct from the emerging specialization in medicine. Psychology, a nonmedical entity, was established as the scholarly discipline for the study of human behavior.

Through the centuries, increasing regard for human life as well as population shifts into larger and larger communities gave impetus to the study and explanation of the plight of individuals who could not communicate. Toward the end of the 19th century, psychoses were recognized as distinct and separate from other aberrant human conditions (Morrison, 1979), while deafness was described as the inability to hear well enough to understand speech (Quigley & Paul, 1984). These early significant developments opened the way to a variety of investigations into those and other behaviors. Neurologists accepted speech, a recognized human behavior as the medium to express mental and emotional intent (Greenblatt & Levinson, 1965). Talking therapy, or psychoanalysis, became a useful mode of treatment for patients whose psychiatric care had formerly depended on hypnosis and drugs. Thus, speech served both as a tool and as content to study. Study of the tool gave clues to the integrity and use of a bioneurological mechanism, whereas study of the content revealed the speaker's experience, emotional status, and cognition. Recognition of the dual value of speech, a basic human behavior, remained near dormant except for the strong movement in study and treatment of deafness in France and England (Moores, 1987).

As the discipline of psychology grew and expanded through the first half of the 20th century, scholarly research on aspects of human behavior produced definitive information concerning human thoughts, feelings, actions, reactions and interactions, norms and differences, and explanatory theories of etiology and prognosis. Also, researchers placed great value on incorporating documentation using the case study technique that was so productive in social work in the late 19th century (Beutler, 1979). The combination of the information generated and the organizational structure of case studies drew aspects of psychology toward the applied sciences with applications foremost in the field of education. Increased research evidence allowed the single discipline of psychology to diversify into a host of specialized fields, including physiological psychology, perception and cognition, human and animal learning, developmental psychology, personality/clinical psychology, social psychology, and educational psychology.

Theories formulated in psychology have been applied to the study of physical, mental, linguistic, and communicative patterns and abilities. Twentieth-century learning theory, linguistic theory, existential and humanistic psychology, as well as medical and environmental discoveries profoundly altered the medical-physical perspectives found in the pre-1900 records of diagnosis and treatment of illness, impairments, and disorders. Perhaps public education of the masses is the greatest experiment that emerged from a common acceptance of the individual's right to access information and the need to know about contemporary society, its governance, its risks, challenges, and rewards.

Greater literacy increased popular knowledge of human conditions and resulted in the eradication of certain superstitions about previously unexplained deviant behavior. The mental illness–wellness dichotomy, inherited from earlier medical approaches to unusual, intolerable behavior, gave way to recognition that a broad range of human behavior may occur without indicating mental illness. Among those behaviors were the communication disorders of deafness, loss of language, and impaired speech, especially stuttering.

Earlier in the 20th century, conscientious teachers of speech had recognized that a small percentage of their students needed special help to alleviate communication disorders and achieve functional communication skills. Those students experienced a level of speech patterns and skills that denied them the expectation of performing at or near the normative level of their peers.

DEVELOPMENT OF THE DISCIPLINE OF COMMUNICATION SCIENCES AND DISORDERS

The descriptor, *communication sciences and disorders*, has come into consistent use only since the 1980s. The term *speech pathology* has been used and recognized for much longer (Guilford, 2003). In the 1924–1925 University of Iowa academic catalogue, the term *speech pathology* was used (Moeller, 1976). In 1927, Robert West and colleagues formalized their commitment to helping those with communication impairments by establishing The American Academy of Speech Correction (Padden, 1970). The academy, based in the educational setting, was founded on two organizational principles:

- Of all the known animals, only humans use symbolic language to express and comprehend cognitive information, use propositional language to deal with abstractions, and use language to create poetry, state scientific principles, or elicit pathos and laughter.
- All human beings have the right to realize their individual potentials.

Before World War II, audiology was not recognized as a separate profession but was identified as a component of *speech correction*. During World War II, Drs. Ray Carhart and Norton Canfield coined the term *audiology* to identify a new science that focused on aural rehabilitation for individuals with war-related hearing loss. The professions of speech pathology and audiology were unified in their efforts to meet the needs of numerous military veterans requiring speech, language, or audiological services. Also, nearly all of the Veteran's Administration hospitals established during this time to serve those injured in the war effort provided rehabilitation programs in speech, language, and hearing.

The 1940s brought dramatic changes in American higher education when thousands of military personnel suddenly returned from World War II. Their needs for training and occupational placement spurred new college and university courses to provide advanced and specialized training to these capable young men and women. The ideal outcome of achieving an occupation through federally funded education forced teachers and professors to revise teaching methods to address almost impossible diversity in huge classes. The diversity among student backgrounds, interests, and abilities was a terrific challenge. Burgeoning interest in advanced study and research in communication disorders, their etiologies, diagnoses, and treatments led to the founding of college and university departments of speech, language, and hearing disorders with names such as Department of Speech and Hearing, Department of Communication Disorders, Communicology, Department of Audiology and Speech Pathology, and Communication Sciences and Disorders. Today, these programs are housed in various colleges within the university setting such as colleges of arts and sciences, education, health sciences, allied health, and public health.

Communication sciences and disorders is a relatively new discipline not offered as a program of study at all colleges and universities. Currently, the Council of Academic Programs in Communication Sciences and Disorders recognizes approximately 250 U.S. graduate programs in the discipline. However, not all of these offer both speech-language pathology and audiology degrees.

After World War II, the discipline's knowledge base continued to grow and major theoretical bases developed. Noam Chomsky (1957, 1968) set the stage for a humanistic approach to language acquisition in his nativist theory of generative transformational grammar, in reaction to B. F. Skinner's behaviorist theory of language acquisition. Each introduced an application of learning and cognitive theory. In behaviorism the child is the recipient and the parent is the active input mechanism. Chomsky, on the other hand, espoused teaching children the rules of language to provide a foundation for their generalized use. That is, the child became an agent in the acquisition and use of language. Later semantic theories insisted that children learn first about meaning and adapt language to express that meaning. Continuing research into language learning has explored many related aspects of language including social learning theory, semantic, cognitive, pragmatic approaches; interactional/conversational approaches; figurative/inferential language; literacy/educational language; and communicative environment.

Another major mid-20th-century contribution to the human services was the work of Carl Rogers (1958). Rogers adapted the term *helping* to connote talking with essentially healthy individuals who need assistance to identify and address problems in their lives. He recognized that some individuals whose behavior he studied could resolve their own difficulties if encouraged to talk logically about the perceived problem and to hypothesize reactions or solutions. In this humanistic approach to psychotherapy, Rogers diverged from the deterministic position of behaviorism and psychiatry. He sought a term for his method that did not contradict the dictum that psychology was strictly the *study* of human behavior and *not* diagnosis or therapeutic management. Rogers and his followers focused on the client as the center of the professional encounter and studied in great depth helper traits and characteristics as a significant portion of the client-professional interaction. This idea had been espoused by the 19th century philosopher, Soren Kierkegaard (1962). Kierkegaard wrote that the clinician, as a person, is the most powerful ingredient in the therapeutic process. Rogers described helping relationships as interpersonal relationships in which one person intends to promote another's growth, development, maturity, improved function, and/or improved coping with life.

The outcome of all of the activity in educational, psychological, and linguistic disciplines fills numerous volumes. We introduce it here to highlight the influence of these disciplines. However, recognizing two public domain outcomes furthers our understanding of the place these specializations hold in the evolution of expertise in speech-language pathology. These outcomes are federal funding for early intervention and treatment of communication disorders among school-age children, those between ages 0 and 21, and the expansion of speech correction to speech-language pathology. Whereas in the early 20th century speech correction had been the purview of teachers of elocution, public speaking, and debate, 100 years later speech-language pathology practitioners must meet the diagnostic and therapeutic needs of clients with communication disorders of all types.

Since that time, other influences (i.e., recognition of need, availability of services, funding resources) have helped develop a widely recognized discipline for preventing and intervening in many handicapping conditions related to disorders of speech, language, and hearing and the physiological mechanisms that enable communication.

It is not surprising that the combination of the three fields of theoretical and practical change in education, psychology, and language, along with public awareness and financial support, have led to elevated expectations of speech-language pathology practitioners. Continuing watchfulness within and around the profession indicates that although professional recognition requires competency in specific areas of speech-language or hearing, career clinical practitioners seek expertise within their specializations.

SPECIALIZATION WITHIN THE DISCIPLINE

Practitioners are influenced by their profession and their discipline. A **profession** is an area of practice. A **discipline** is an area of study or specialization of study. The discipline of **communication sciences and disorders (CSD)** encompasses study of the human communication process, the science of human communication, breakdowns in the processes of human communication (referred to as communication differences or disorders), and the efficacy of the applied disciplinary practices. Communication sciences and disorders represent three primary professions: speech, language, and hearing science; audiology; and speech-language pathology. In addition, the discipline includes related areas of practice. These areas deal with deafness and deaf education and include professionals who develop and apply educational and rehabilitative techniques for individuals with severe and profound hearing impairments (Guilford, 2003).

Early pioneers in establishing the professional discipline of speech-language pathology came from postgraduate training programs in psychology, education, medical science, and linguistics. Many brought with them a deep and abiding interest in communication disorders based on personal experience of living with a speech disorder. As undergraduate and postgraduate curricula developed within the communication disorders specialization, frequent and repeated selections of materials, methods, programs, and their applications drew on these and other scholarly fields. The blending of knowledge through research and clinical application in diagnosis and treatment of communication disorders produced modified theory and practice that better suited client needs in this narrowly defined segment of human behavior. Early focus on the sound stream humans produce as speech led investigators to consider the etiologies of the disorders. Many theories of psychology were adapted to explain **dysfluency** as well as to construct systems for treating the stutterer. Gradually, not only linguists and scholars of deaf culture but also the hearing world began to recognize American Sign Language as a separate and distinct language (Bellugi & Klima, 1972). An even farther-reaching progression, recognition of neurological bases of language as well as perception and production of speech, has become a fundamental standard in the practice and research of speech-language pathology. Currently, adaptation, development, and inclusion of instrumentation, technology, and research from other disciplines further enhance the practice of speech-language pathology.

The importance of speech-language pathology services has been enhanced by public demand and heightened awareness of communicative needs of constituents in the national political arena. During the later decades of the 20th century, federal funding for support of services and for research became available in the United States with passage of legislation that spelled out rights of school-age children. Other congressional decisions established comprehensive programs on aging.

IMPACT OF EDUCATIONAL, LEGISLATIVE, AND MEDICAL ISSUES

Educational legislative issues have had strong impact on the profession, beginning in the 1970s and 1980s when initiatives generally focused on children 3 to 21 years of age. See Table 2.1 for a summary of federally mandated legislative changes.

TABLE 2.1   Legislative Mandates That Have Influenced the Profession

Year	Title of Legislative Act	Significance
1975	P.L. 94-142	Increased service to children with communication disorders 6–21 years of age.
1986	P.L. 99-457 Education for the Handicapped Act	Increased age range of children who are served from ages 3–5 and 6–21.
	P.L. 102-119 (Amended P.L. 99-457) became known as Part H	Part H mandated that ALL states provide services for 3–5-year-olds with special needs.
1990	Reauthorization of Education for the Handicapped Act into Individuals with Disabilities Education Act (IDEA)	Later reauthorized again and moved Part H to Part C.
2004	Reauthorization of IDEA	Strengthened the role of Naturalistic Environments.
2005	No Child Left Behind	Designed to strengthen the academic performance of students whose schools are failing them. Only qualified schools are those receiving Title I funds (low-income schools).

School systems established preschool programs and educationally relevant programs for older children as the initial result of Public Law 94-142. This law produced enormous growth in numbers of school-age children served in the schools because their communication disorders were designated *educationally relevant*. The treatment must have a positive impact on the child's ability to learn and meet educational objectives. During this time, school districts were mandated to serve children ages 6 to 21 and encouraged to serve children ages 3 to 5. In 1986, an amendment to the act, Public Law 99-457, became known as **Education for the Handicapped Act.** This act was later amended as Public Law 102-119 and became know as Part H. **Part H** mandated that all states provide services for children ages 3 to 5 with special needs.

In 1990, the Education for the Handicapped Act was reauthorized under the **Individuals with Disabilities Education Act (IDEA)** and it was again reauthorized under the same name but with the services for infants and toddlers moved from Part H to **Part C.** This reauthorization strengthened the role of naturalistic environments and families and boosted the requirements for transition planning between Part C programs and **Part B** programs—those for children ages 3–21. It should also be noted that **naturalistic environments** were defined as those in which children of the same age, but without disabilities, would typically be found. Naturalistic environments have typically been interpreted as services provided in the home or in a child-care center for *typically developing* children (Billeaud, 1998). The 2004 version of IDEA contains language to (1) study the relationship between environmental factors and developmental disabilities; (2) cap the amount of fees that attorneys can charge for due-process cases; (3) allow the **individualized educational plan (IEP)** to follow transient students; and (4) reduce the amount of paperwork required for implementation (NOMA, 2004). IDEA was reauthorized on December 3, 2004. Details of the reauthorization of Public Law 108-446, **Individuals with Disabilities Education Improvement Act of 2004** may be viewed on the *Federal Register* website. The American Speech-Language-Hearing Association link to this website at http://www.ASHA.org.

No Child Left Behind is the nation's most recent initiative to increase the academic performance of children who are attending schools that are failing to prepare children to make **adequate yearly progress (AYP).** In this program, each state sets standards for academic achievement in its schools. Schools receiving federal Title I funds that fail to meet the state's goals are designated as needing improvement and must notify parents. The full impact of this program on the speech-language pathology profession is unclear at this time. The program is strongly literacy and math based, but will likely also involve more speech-language pathologists through the language-based components of these two areas. (http://www.ed.gov/nclb/landing.jhtml). Some speculate that the federal government may lack sufficient funds to implement fully this program throughout the United States. This program will continue to develop throughout the next decade.

An additional governmental influence on professional practice has been requirements for reimbursement. Reimbursement now involves coding that is essential for third-party billing (e.g., insurance, Medicare, Medicaid, state funding). The billing codes identify diagnostic and treatment procedures, client diagnosis, and essential devices or supplies and equipment. The regulatory body for the health-care services coding system is the Centers for Medicare and Medicaid Services (CMS). Additional legislation effecting billing and patient records was established through the **Health Insurance Portability and Accountability Act (HIPAA).** The three current coding systems are as follows:

➤ Current Procedural Terminology (CPT)
  http://www.ama-assn.org/ama/pub/category/3113.html

➤ Healthcare Common Procedures Coding System (HCPCS)
  http://www.cms.hhs.gov/medicare/hcpcs

➤ International Classification of Diseases, 9th edition, Clinical Modification (ICD-9-CM)
  http://www.cdc.gov/ichs/about/otheract/icd9/abticd10.htm

ASHA provides the practitioner with information and support related to coding through frequently asked questions (FAQs) for audiologists and speech-language pathologists on their website (http://www.ASHA.org).

With increasing longevity across the population and a rise in numbers of neurogenic communication disorders among the elderly, communication sciences has expanded attention to brain function in language loss, acquired speech disorders, and swallowing disorders. These studies necessarily examined the outcomes of genetics, wear and tear, pathology, or trauma. Initially targeting the elderly, neurogenics gradually took on a global perspective to include developmental as well as traumatic disorders in children and young adults.

As speech-language pathology became more individuated and client specific and as the scope of practice evolved, the profession also evolved. Today, clinical practice occurs in many settings, including schools, hospitals, rehabilitation facilities, clinics, and private practices. Clinical practitioners who stay current must keep up a broad-based knowledge of the health-care system, the constraints of illness/wellness on the patient/client/family, and the implications for reimbursement by third-party payers who wield considerable decision-making influence over patient/client treatment. The saturation of speech-language pathology with clearly defined characteristics and required services marks the discipline as one of the continually growing human services fields.

SUMMARY

Speech-language pathology has evolved as a human services profession through convergence of principles from many other human services disciplines. The profession has primarily developed in the mid-20th century to the present. The universal acceptance of human communication as a basic right and need of all people led to incorporation of discoveries from a variety of professions. This incorporation of various areas is attributed to those who could see their shared knowledge as valuable through all levels of community endeavor from individual need to federal consensus for funding and support.

THOUGHTS FOR EXPLORATION

1. Compare modern diagnosis and treatment of communication disorders with perceptions of handicapping conditions across time.
2. What impact did World War II have on the discipline of communication sciences and disorders?
3. Discuss Kierkegaard's 19th-century dictum that "the clinician as a person is the most powerful ingredient in the therapeutic process."

REFERENCES

American Personnel and Guidance Association. (1965). *Ethical standards handbook.* Washington, DC: Author.

Bellugi, U., & Klima, E. (1972). The roots of language in the sign talk of the deaf. *Psychology Today, 6,* 61–78.

Beutler, L. E. (1979). Values, beliefs, religion, and the persuasive influence of psychotherapy. *Psychotherapy Theory, Research and Practice, 16,* 432–440.

Billeaud, F. P. (1998). *Communication disorders in infants and toddlers: Assessment and intervention* (2nd ed.). Woburn, MA: Butterworth-Heinemann.

Chomsky, N. (1957). *Syntactic structures.* The Hague: Mouton.

Chomsky, N. (1968). *Language and the mind.* New York: Harcourt, Brace and World.

Cole, L. (1982). *Helping*. Toronto: Butterworth.

Crouch, A. (1997). *Inside counseling: Becoming and being a professional*. Thousand Oaks, CA: Sage.

Egan, G. (2002). *The skilled helper: A problem-management and opportunity development approach to helping* (7th ed.). Pacific Grove, CA: Brooks/Cole.

Emener, W. G., & Darrow, M. A. (1991). *Career exploration in human services*. Springfield, IL: Charles C Thomas.

Greenblatt, M., & Levinson, J. L. (1965). Mental hospitals. In Benjamin B. Wolman (Ed.), *Handbook of clinical psychology* (pp. 1343–1359). New York: McGraw-Hill.

Guilford, A. (2003). Communication sciences and disorders. In M. A. Richard & W. G. Emener (Eds.), *I'm a people person: A guide to human services professions*. Springfield, IL: Charles C Thomas.

Kierkegaard, S. (1962). *The point of view for my work as an author: A report of history*. New York: Harper Torchbooks.

Mill, J. S. (1975). *On liberty*. New York: Norton. (Original work published in 1859).

Moeller, D. (1976). *Speech pathology and audiology: Iowa organization of a discipline*. Iowa City: University of Iowa Press.

Moores, D. (1987). *Educating the deaf: Psychology, principles, and practices*. Boston: Houghton Mifflin.

Morrison, J. K. (1979). A consumer-oriented approach to psychotherapy. *Psychotherapy: Theory, Research, and Practice, 16*, 381–384.

National Outcomes Measurement System. (2004). *ASHA Leader, 9*, (11), 3.

Padden, E. P. (1970). *A history of the American Speech and Hearing Association: 1925 to 1958*. Washington, DC: American Speech and Hearing Association.

Perry, P. A. (1996). *Opportunities in mental health careers*. Chicago, IL: VGM Career Horizons.

Quigley, S. P., & Paul P. V. (1984). *Deafness*. San Diego: College-Hill Press.

Richard, M. A., & Emener, W. G. (Eds.). (2003). *I'm a people person: A guide to human service professions*. Springfield, IL: Charles C Thomas.

Rogers, C. (1958). The characteristics of a helping relationship. *Personnel and Guidance Journal, 37*, 6–16.

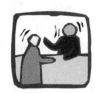

CHAPTER 3

Expertise in Speech-Language Pathology

Factors of Expertise Each of the five major elements of the model of expertise is designated as a factor that includes specific indicators (knowledge, skills, and traits) related to the development of expertise.

INTRODUCTION

Expertise is a conceptual framework for distinguishing levels of skill and knowledge in the profession. As such, we can identify, observe, measure, and describe expertise. In doing so, we formulate a general theory of expertise and define the conditions under which it exists. Many theories of expertise have been developed in various disciplines (Sternberg & Grigorenko, 2003). Expertise in speech-language pathology is revealed in the knowledge, skills, personal/interpersonal characteristics, and practice of the clinician. These are considered indicators of expertise. Research findings confirm that the concept of expertise exists and that expertise is essential to professional practice. In addition, research findings suggest that speech-language pathology expertise is a broad concept that may be represented by five factors and associated indicators (Graham, 1998). Although beginning professionals enter the field with minimal competence, expertise may be a professional goal that includes a path for continuing professional growth.

THE FACTORS OF EXPERTISE

According to Graham (1998) and Graham and Guilford (2000) expertise in speech-language pathology practice is represented by these five factors:

- *Factor 1—Interpersonal Skills* include personal traits and all aspects of interactive skills.
- *Factor 2—Professional Skills* are acquired and regulated behaviors that are discipline specific and indicate an individual's compliance with standards, codes, and responsibilities encompassed by the profession.
- *Factor 3—Problem-Solving Skills* are cognitive abilities to quickly recognize unique or challenging situations and to proceed readily with efficient, effective, and satisfying resolution or management.

- *Factor 4—Technical Skills* are derived from knowledge and practical experience gained through use of materials, technology, techniques, and procedures learned during professional education or continuing education and selectively applied.
- *Factor 5—Knowledge and Experience* the individual clinician amasses over time are the products of study in discipline-based curricula in higher education; conscientious attention to practice with a variety of clients/patients with similar diagnoses; consistent review of current research; and continuing education to maintain certification and professional license(s).

These factors provide a comprehensive overview of the concept of expertise as it is recognized in the profession. Simply stated, speech-language pathologists have high expectations of professionals recognized as experts. The list of skills and traits that exemplify expertise is extensive and the comprehensive model of expertise presented here represents the standard.

Although the list of skills and traits is lengthy and comprehensive, these may be grouped using statistical methods according to the five factors and according to importance between and within the factors. In general, the rank order within factors is not significant in degree. However, the following are generally agreed on:

- A solid base of knowledge gained through education and experience is a critical basis for developing expertise.
- Technical skills must be taught and practiced across time.
- As observed in the research from other disciplines, the ability to solve problems quickly and effectively differentiates novice from expert.
- Professional skills are specific to the profession and may reflect individual initiative in achieving professional development.
- Regardless of levels of competence in all other areas, interpersonal skills have the most readily observable impact on success in the practice of the profession.

Becoming an expert is determined by the mastery of interpersonal skills, professional skills, problem-solving skills, technical skills, and the acquisition and judicial use of knowledge and experience. Within each of these basic factors are found unique features observable in student and novice clinicians, as well as experts. Over time, advanced skills, knowledge, and practices emerge with increased involvement in the discipline. We believe each feature of these five basic factors has relative importance to demonstrating expertise. The interaction among the individual's traits, behaviors, and skills, as well as the clinician's degree of competence in each area reflects the clinician's progress in developing expertise.

Expertise develops along a continuum, although not necessarily in a linear fashion. Expertise in the helping professions is not attained only by accumulating skills and years of experience (Jennings, 1996). Every human service profession has individuals who studied all the appropriate academic curricula and have years of experience but have failed to attain recognition as experts in their fields. Thus, it is possible to become an experienced nonexpert (Sternberg & Horvath, 1995). Developing expertise, however, is a highly desirable goal that professionals can achieve through an accessible process that can be pursued and monitored.

It follows that expertise in speech-language pathology is discernable and obtainable (Cornett & Chabon, 1988). Expertise includes the requisite knowledge, specialized skills, and techniques often attested to by education and certification requirements. The recognition of a continuum of expertise provides incentive and encouragement for the professional throughout the process. Seeing development of expertise as a professional challenge reflects this continuum and offers a pathway for professional growth. This description suggests the need for an approach to expertise that is responsive and fluid rather than exclusionary and static.

THE COMPONENTS OF THE FACTORS OF EXPERTISE

Interpersonal skills describe the personal attitude, manner, and style of the professional as an individual. This factor tends to provide a foundation and essential element to the model of expertise that distinguishes the expert from other professionals within the discipline. It includes many indicators described by previous research (Chermak & Scheuerle, 1996; Scheuerle, 1992) as essential in the helping professions. Its mature development may also often account for the difference between the expert and the experienced nonexpert. This foundational factor is an important feature of the professional practitioner because it is *what the preprofessional brings* to the process of education and training. Evaluating interpersonal skills requires only a client or patient's response rather than their intentional, informed assessment of a professional's knowledge and skills. Those who know little of the profession's technical aspects can easily identify a clinician who has well-developed interpersonal skills as compared to a clinician who lacks them. Clients/patients, when responding to quality assurance surveys, are often more influenced by "how" the clinician acted or performed than by "what" he or she did for them. Of course, strong interpersonal skills may initially mask weakness in other factors of expertise. As a result, interpersonal skills may distinguish an expert speech-language pathologist when supported by exceptional performance in the remaining factors.

This factor includes features that, if developed and consciously used, promote excellence and enhance performance. These characteristics represent both the clinician's personal and professional impact on the diagnostic or therapeutic process. Researchers have described interpersonal skills as essential to expertise in a helping profession (Richard & Emener, 2003). All aspects of one's daily and professional life display personal traits and interpersonal skills that include variations and combinations of the individual and multiple features. However, interpersonal skills alone do not make an expert clinician.

Desired features of Interpersonal Skills are listed in Table 3.1. They clearly reflect aspects of the individual that relate specifically to *how* one interacts with others in a professional, caring manner. For example, the ability to actively listen, show cultural sensitivity, demonstrate empathy, and exhibit honesty in a nondefensive manner are all essential behaviors during interviews, diagnostic sessions, or treatment procedures.

Within the factor, three divisions of the features of interpersonal skills include verbal/nonverbal interactions, personality traits, and social and cultural disposition. Specific features related to observable verbal/nonverbal interactions include active listening, body language, and reinforcing behaviors. These features are reflected in the way the clinician relates to the client/patient and other significant individuals. The majority of the features may be attributed to personality and include cooperation, enthusiasm, flexibility, friendliness, honesty, humility, intuition, nondefensiveness, open-minded attitude, patience, positive attitude, self-motivation, sincerity, tactfulness, and trustworthiness. Although we consider these personality traits generally positive, their purposeful application in the clinical context indicates ability to self-monitor and interact in a positive, constructive manner. The remaining features convey social and cultural disposition. These features include acceptance, cultural sensitivity, empathy, respect for others and tolerance. Development and application of these traits in a professional setting allows the clinician to make appropriate referrals, meet the needs of clients/patients and caregivers, and work effectively with persons from backgrounds and cultures different from their own.

The features presented in Table 3.1 often affect the effort put forth to become an expert in an increasingly diverse population. Beginning clinicians may find objectively and accurately identifying their own interpersonal skills inventory a challenge. Issues of maturity, ability to accept suggestions, defensiveness, extent of experience, and lack of awareness of future benefits may inhibit progress in this area. Aspects of

TABLE 3.1   Selected Features of Interpersonal Skills

Acceptance	Willing and favorable tolerance of individuals and their behavior.
Active listening	Alert attending to verbal and nonverbal messages with nonverbal reinforcement.
Appropriate body language	Posture and movement commensurate with communication partner and setting.
Cooperation	Helpful and supportive behaviors.
Cultural sensitivity	Knowledge, awareness, and concern for customs, beliefs, and practices different from one's own.
Dependability	Reliability, steadiness, steadfastness.
Empathy	The ability to experience feelings similar to those of someone else.
Enthusiasm	Eagerness and interest in the action or situation.
Flexibility	Willingness and ability to change in response to changing circumstances.
Friendliness	Positive acceptance of and interaction with others.
Honesty	Sincerity, truthfulness, integrity.
Humility	Absence of pride or self-assertion.
Intuition	Instinctive perception of the behaviors of others.
Nondefensive Manner	Freedom from the need to explain or enlarge on one's thoughts or feelings.
Open-mindedness	Pursuit of experiences and knowledge with acceptance and without bias.
Patience	Calm tolerance of delay, confusion, or inefficiency.
Positive attitude	Optimistic outlook in expectations.
Reinforcing	Encouraging a behavior to continue.
Respectful	Expressing esteem for someone else.
Self-motivation	Inherent ability to have ongoing goals.
Sincerity	Genuine, straightforward, and truthful.
Tactfulness	Diplomatic and discreet action.
Tolerance	Open-minded and forbearing demeanor.
Trustworthiness	Dependability and reliability.

one's personal makeup may be among the most difficult to self-evaluate and modify, and yet they can have a significant impact on success and self-satisfaction. A personal inventory or list of skills already mastered and those to be addressed directly during professional development is beneficial. Appendix A provides an inventory for self-evaluation. Experts use such inventories as tools for maximizing effective delivery of services. They demonstrate conscious use of skills and minimize nonproductive behaviors and traits.

Professional skills represent advanced knowledge and clinical practice. These indicators represent advanced skills (beyond minimal competence) as they relate to day-to-day service and management of professional responsibilities. The indicators relate generally to professional conduct and specifically to the roles and responsibilities unique to each practice setting.

These skills represent all of the planning and work that ensure treatment efficacy, service delivery, and communication support for clients/patients. Professional behaviors in speech-language pathology practice resemble those of other helping professions. That is, through all the features listed in Table 3.2, we readily see that the clinician's professional behavior addresses responsibilities to the consumer, to colleagues, to the workplace, and to the discipline as a whole. The meaning of each feature is both general as it relates to professional conduct and specific as it relates to the roles and responsibilities unique to the demands of each practice setting.

As stated earlier, this factor represents features that relate to the clinical context/work setting, to the community at large, and to the profession. Features related to the clinical context include the professional's ability to supervise (staff, colleagues,

TABLE 3.2   Selected Features of Professional Skills

Ability to supervise	Possessing knowledge and skills for overseeing and mentoring the clinical behavior of others.
Awareness of community	Mindful of available resources and reciprocal behaviors of other professionals.
Compliance with licensure, rules, and regulations	Awareness of and compliance with state, federal, and professional association mandates.
Conducting or using relevant research	Becoming a critical thinker and consumer of research relevant to best practices for clinical services.
Consultation and collaboration	Interacting with other helping professionals to plan for effective clinical practice.
Data collection and dissemination	Carefully gathering information from all sources and distributing it to others accurately and without delay for the client's welfare.
Discharge planning	Effective methods of transfer, referral, or termination of client for clinical services.
Record keeping	Management of confidential clinical documents in an organized and retrievable manner that comply with current standards of care.
Resource management	Budgeting financial resources.
Specialization	Acquiring advanced knowledge relevant to the clinical practice for specific disorders.
Utilization of payment methods for health care	Using private, public, and third-party payer coverage of health care.

clinicians in training, clinical fellows), to conduct and use relevant research, to keep useful records and documentation, to effectively manage resources (finances, facility, materials, personnel), and to use appropriate payment or reimbursement methods. All of these are crucial to successful delivery of services and facility operation. Features that relate to the community at large include an awareness of characteristics, demographics, and unique aspects of the practice's geographic area; ability to consult and collaborate with others within and outside of the discipline; ability to collect, interpret, use, and disseminate clinical data; and attention to the requirements for discharge planning to achieve successful transitions for clients/patients. Finally, several features relate specifically to the profession of speech-language pathology and its associated professional organizations and governing bodies. These include compliance with requirements for certification, professional license, and state and national rules and regulations; and development of a specialization within an ever-expanding profession.

The ongoing demands of maintaining professional status and a respected standing in the community requires the practitioner to participate in all the tasks that ensure that recognition continues. The essential tasks include but are not limited to client case management, site maintenance, monitoring fiscal responsibility, ready communication with colleagues who may serve the same population, advocacy with colleagues within the profession and in other professions, profession advancement through clinical research, and active participation in professional associations.

Features of **problem-solving skills** listed in Table 3.3 represent decision-making activities in the clinical role. The indicators in this factor tend to relate directly to outcomes and lend themselves to measurement and correlation with treatment outcomes. These skills are critical from the moment of meeting a new client/patient to dismissal following treatment. Problem solving requires the best of personal insight, technical ability, broad-based education, applied knowledge, and a keen literate interest in research to underlie service to each individual. For the client/patient to achieve effective and efficient progress in treatment, the clinician must

- Identify the multiple aspects and implications of the client's communication disorder
- Analyze and set priorities among elements of the problem(s)
- Explore realistically the effects and implications of the existing problem

TABLE 3.3 Selected Features of Problem-Solving Skills

Case management	Attention to details of time, effort, outcomes, and planning for the client.
Confidence	Assurance in self-knowledge and ability.
Decision making	Rational analysis and conclusion within a flexible frame of reference.
Ethical conduct	Conscientious observance of the spectrum of communication disorders to which training and experience apply; working within scope of practice.
Experience	Ability to carry over valuable lessons learned through effort.
Follow-through	Ongoing interest and effort after an assignment or determination of need.
Good judgment	Rational-emotive balance in drawing conclusions about client care.
Making referrals	Assignment of client to identified colleagues or other professionals with specialized knowledge.
Observant	Ongoing awareness of client behavior, environment, and interaction.
Part-to-whole analysis	Synthesis/coordination of details (parts) to arrive at a total picture.
Professional communication	Effective formal exchange of oral and written information between clients, colleagues, and caregivers.
Time management	Effective and efficient use of time.
Treatment efficacy	Applications of selected techniques to facilitate achievement of anticipated goals.
Use of task modification techniques	Ability to alter procedures, strategies, or techniques when called for.

- Synthesize potential responses to client needs and colleague inquiries concerning the client
- Establish a reasonable client prognosis and plan of intervention
- Identify and obtain equipment, materials, and consultations needed to complete the treatment
- Utilize current research to implement evidence-based intervention
- Procure reimbursement for services

The features of problem-solving skills are responsive to continued practice and focused learning. As a result, these skills may improve across time given concentrated effort and emphasis.

Some features set standards for professional conduct and represent how others see the professional such as acting with confidence, ethical conduct, being observant, and being experienced. Other features specifically relate to how clinicians carry out their duties and responsibilities: case load management, effective follow-through, use of good judgment, making appropriate referrals, professional communication style, and effective time management. These features affect productivity, effectiveness, and success in meeting client/patient needs in professional practice. The remaining features of problem solving represent specific strategies implemented to maximize outcomes and professional achievement through conscious decision-making processes, part-to-whole analysis of situations, application of evidence-based practice to achieve treatment efficacy, and the use of task modification techniques and task hierarchy when planning and implementing services.

Examination of this factor of expertise reflects previous research in expert–novice differences (National Outcomes Measurement System [NOMS], 2003). Like interpersonal skills, problem-solving skills may be inherent to the individual. However, they may also be acquired through practice, experience, and direct learning.

The features of **technical skills** are unique to speech-language pathology as a discipline and to speech-language pathologists as members of the profession and specific in their relationship to assessment and treatment. The specific meaning and application of each feature may vary in relation to different practice settings and treatment protocols.

All features in this factor relate to evaluating and treating diverse disorders in a variety of clinical settings. They deal with selection and use of materials, instrumentation, and techniques; interpretation of responses, behaviors, and conditions; formulation of recommendations and future course(s) of action; and the ability to engage in communication (spoken and written) in a professional style and manner.

As we see from the features cited in Table 3.4, preprofessionals learn technical skills in classes/structured educational activities and as they apply knowledge and skills during supervised clinical experience. The practicing speech-language pathologist continues to develop and improve technical skill through continuing education, shadowing (observing another professional during their daily schedule of service delivery), and working with skilled speech-language pathologists recognized for their expertise and areas of specialization. Professionals also attend conferences, read current research publications, and participate in professional associations. These are essential to effective clinical management, but alone they do not signify true expertise in speech-language pathology.

Technical skills of the speech-language pathologist incorporate all the knowledge and its application to the use of materials, tools, equipment, methodologies, techniques, and strategies necessary to ongoing evaluation and treatment for each client regardless of the communication disorder, its severity, complexity, or duration. The competent and flexible clinician uses documented evidence garnered by conscientious observation to introduce modifications to plans and protocols when indicated by special circumstances of the client.

Knowledge and experience represent access to basic information primary to the novice-to-expert continuum. Knowledge here means the combination of content/theoretical

TABLE 3.4   Selected Features of Technical Skills

Formulation of appropriate recommendations	Analysis of data and observations that leads to formulation of objectives and goals.
Implementation of diagnostic tools and procedures	Selection and administration of protocols that effectively identify and assess the communication disorder(s).
Interpretation of test results and procedures	Analysis of data from tests and observations and case history information that lead to the design of an effective treatment plan.
Oral communication skills	The ability to present relevant information through clear, jargon-free speech that provides an appropriate clinical model.
Selection of appropriate tools and procedures	The ability to knowledgeably choose from the broad spectrum of available tools and procedures those that will best address the client's condition.
Task analysis	The ability to separate a given task into its component parts and identify strengths and weaknesses in performance.
Task selection and implementation	Matching the treatment design to the skill level and potential of the client.
Treatment implementation	The ability to introduce and follow through with a planned program design.
Treatment planning	Based on the results of tests and observations, the ability to select and sequence tasks and experiences that will create effective change.
Written communication skills	Effectively communicating results and recommendations to clients and referral sources through professional writing.

TABLE 3.5 Selected Features of Knowledge and Experience

Academic course work	The prescribed sequence of study that will deliver the knowledge and skills required for ASHA certification.
Active learner	Taking initiative in mastering new knowledge.
Advanced or specialized knowledge base	A level of understanding that exceeds the basic competencies and moves the individual toward becoming an expert.
Continuing education	The continuation of learning experiences under the auspices of approved teachers or trainers. Required for certification and licensure.
Familiarity with applicable Codes of Ethics	Understanding the range of behaviors that fall within the scope of practice defined by profession ethical standards and the Code of Ethics.
Field work experience: internship/externship	Educational experiences in which the student applies clinical skills in various off-campus settings under the supervision of experienced, certified clinicians.
Knowledge of research methods	Understanding the principles and applications of research methodology that document clinical experience and provide evidence of benefits of treatment.
Lifelong learning	A term often applied to the need and desire to participate in perpetual inquiry and continuing education.
Practicum experience	Clinical education and training during a program of study that provide opportunities to initiate and carry out treatment and evaluation while under the direct supervision of a qualified professional.

knowledge and experiential/applied knowledge of the discipline. In addition, this factor addresses not only the basic academic foundations of speech-language pathology but also advanced and specialized information. This demonstrates ongoing professional growth through continued learning. Knowledge and experience includes the features that are seen in Table 3.5.

These features represent the foundational cumulative knowledge and experience bank for the beginning professional and the advanced, specialized knowledge and experience for the developing expert. They represent the ongoing, lifelong, proactive act of learning grounded in the profession's ethical code.

The clinical practitioner gathers knowledge and experience through curricula of accredited graduate programs in colleges and universities. The evolving scope of practice across the discipline requires novices to have a broad knowledge base. As the knowledge base increases, the practitioner faces the challenge of learning more about all types of communication disorders experienced across cultures and ethnic groups and in different contexts. As knowledge and experience increase, each practitioner has the potential and opportunity to collect data vital to professional advancement.

Both professionals and the profession have an ongoing need for clinical research. After all, the clinical practice of speech-language pathology is both the method of service delivery and the source of scientific information on which the profession is based.

RELATIVE VALUE AND INTERACTION OF THE FIVE FACTORS OF SPEECH-LANGUAGE PATHOLOGY EXPERTISE

All five factors of expertise in speech-language pathology are critical to the development of expertise within the profession. Further, they have an order of importance in the demonstration of expertise. The essential features of expertise that emerge from examination of each factor are unique as they relate to effectiveness of clinical services and outcomes for clients/patients. To be considered an expert, the clinician must demonstrate exceptional performance in each area. No one factor or set of features will distinguish an individual as an expert. An obvious interaction between factors necessitates excellence across all factors. However, it is unclear how many features within each factor the individual must demonstrate to achieve such recognition. It is accepted that the expert speech-language pathologist effectively and frequently uses self-monitoring skills in the form of self-evaluation (ASHA, 2003) to further professional development.

It is also important to recognize that expertise is not a static entity. Expertise develops over time as a function of experience developing on a continuum. Diversity within the profession across the scope of practice and the variability among practice settings presents a significant challenge to identifying and defining expertise. Figure 3.1 illustrates the relationship and interdependence of the five factors of expertise as a pyramid with successive layers representing the features of each factor. The mass of each ascending tier of the pyramid reflects the emphasis placed on the factors by consensus definition of expertise in speech-language pathology (Graham, 1998). The features of each tier interact with others within and among the five factors. The foundation of expertise lies in personal traits and interpersonal skills that include personal and professional attributes of behavior. These features, found in most helping professions, support, permeate, and shape the upper layers. Viewed according to their relative importance in development of expertise, the strata of the pyramid suggest both the weight of each factor and the power of the features within each factor to affect overall acquisition of expertise.

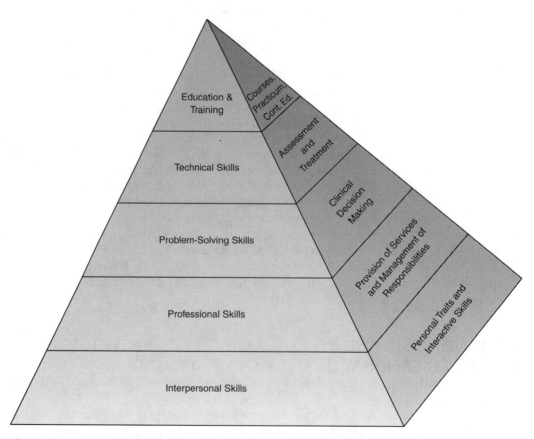

Figure 3.1 A Model of Clinical Expertise

Additionally, the upper three tiers of the pyramid include factors of expertise that, when combined, are a composite of *professional competencies*. That is, the pyramid emphasizes the critical place of interpersonal skills and professional skills as ability banks that support and pervade the individualized application of all the features of professional competencies. Strengths in all the features and in their blended application lead to recognition of expertise. Weakness in any one or more of the strata or even among the features within one stratum diminishes the composite whole essential to achieve the goal of expertise. When weaknesses emerge in clinician conduct, those features can be identified and addressed individually.

Expertise in speech-language pathology is distinct from expertise in any other helping profession or discipline. Although we expect similarity among certain traits and actions of all helping professions, expert performance in one discipline does not automatically transfer to another discipline. Certainly, specialized knowledge and technical skills would remain pertinent to the original profession.

The apex of the pyramid emphasizes specialized education and training as the focal point that separates the speech-language pathologist from practitioners of other helping professions. In each helping profession a well-developed bank of knowledge and lifelong learning are essential elements of expertise as represented in specialized knowledge and experience (Elstein, 1988). Expertise in each helping profession depends heavily on a well-organized store of discipline-specific knowledge that invites retrieval and application to new situations. A strong knowledge base and a commitment to lifelong learning are fundamental assumptions when describing expertise within the profession of speech-language pathology. Creative learning witnessed in clinical practice involves more than clinical competence. The mastery and specialization of technical and problem-solving skills reflect ongoing development of expertise. A commitment to learning and expansion of correlative understanding is important, as is conscientious self-evaluation.

SUMMARY

The broad, multifaceted nature of expertise in the profession of speech-language pathology makes its acquisition a comprehensive process. Expertise is not merely the sum of knowledge acquired, years of experience, and skills mastered; it is an ongoing process molded by the traits and abilities of each individual speech-language pathologist. Expertise is an inner-driven synergy that enables the practitioner to blend the art and the science of the profession to yield the expert.

THOUGHTS FOR EXPLORATION

1. What are the five factors of expertise in speech-language pathology derived from the research of Graham and Guilford?
2. What is the meaning of the following statement?: "The recent graduate in speech-language pathology is a novice in clinical practice."
3. Of the 24 features of interpersonal skills, which best represent your strengths? Which should be targeted for development and improvement?
4. Review the features of technical skills in terms of your clinical observation and experience, and describe the role of each in the treatment process.
5. Why is the following statement true?: "Knowledge and skills are expected to increase throughout a career."

REFERENCES

American Speech-Language-Hearing Association. (2003, November). (Tech. Rep. Draft). Rockville, MD: Author.

Chermak, G. D. & Scheuerle, J. (1996). Designing and Teaching University Courses in Counseling and Collaboration. *ASHA*, 1996 Convention, Seattle, Washington.

Cornett, B. S., & Chabon, S. S. (1988). *The clinical practice of speech-language pathology.* Columbus, OH: Merrill.

Elstein, A. S. (1988). Cognitive processes in clinical inference and decision making. In D. C. Turk & P. Salovey (Eds.), *Reasoning, inference, and judgment in clinical psychology* (pp. 17–50). New York: Free Press.

Graham, S. V. (1998). *Quality treatment indicators: A model for clinical expertise in speech-language pathology.* Doctoral dissertation, University of South Florida, Tampa.

Graham, S. V. & Guilford A. M. (2000, November). *Beyond competence: Development of a model of clinical expertise.* American Speech-Language-Hearing Association annual conference, Washington, DC.

Jennings, L. (1996). *Personal characteristics of master therapists.* Morris, MN: University of Minnesota.

National Outcomes Measurement System (2003). *ASHA Leader, 9*(11), 3.

Richard, M. A., & Emener, W. G. (2003). *I'm a people person: A guide to human service professions.* Springfield, IL.

Scheuerle, J. (1992). *Counseling in Speech-Language Pathology and Audiology.* New York: Macmillan Publishing Company.

Sternberg, R. J., & Grigorenko, E. L. (2003). *The psychology of abilities, competencies, and expertise.* Cambridge, U.K.: Cambridge University Press.

Sternberg, R. J., & Horvath, J. A. (1995). A prototype view of expert teaching. *Educational Researcher, 24*(6), 9–17.

CHAPTER 4

Novice to Expert: A Continuum

Novice A clinician who has completed and mastered basic and advanced educational and clinical experiences and is completing the requirements of the fellowship year and other requirements for the Certificate of Clinical Competence (CCC), certification(s), and licensure, if applicable. Typically, this individual is in the early years of practice.

Expert A recognized authority who frequently has specialized and who has obtained basic, advanced, and continuing education and training. Through skill development in knowledge and experience, technical skills, problem-solving skills, professional skills, and interpersonal skills becomes known and recognized as an expert often within a specialized scope of practice and employment setting.

INTRODUCTION

The emerging focus on expertise in speech-language pathology practice relates to many social, political, and professional movements. These movements have prompted the profession and professionals to adjust to an expanding scope of practice and new requirements for knowledge, skills, and competencies. Recognition of speech-language pathology as an autonomous profession by providers and payers is essential to protect and promote the scope of practice. Without recognition, the profession and the quality of services its members provide are threatened on many fronts. Similarly, regard for the services provided ensures that quality services are made available and sustained in a variety of settings for individuals with communication disorders. That is, the valuation of the profession, its members, and the services provided is a reciprocal interaction between participants. Likewise, consumer expectations ensure that professionals meet standards of education and training, standards of practice, standards of ethical conduct within an identified scope of practice, and standards of continuing education.

In an effort to systematize and standardize academic and clinical preparation of novice clinicians, the American Speech-Language-Hearing Association (ASHA) established criteria for accreditation of university training programs and criteria for graduate students in speech-language pathology who pursue and attain the Certificate of Clinical Competence (CCC). Students must meet these standards-based criteria to be certified as qualified to practice speech-language pathology in most settings. These standards are further promoted by ASHA's 2004 continuing education requirement to maintain the CCC. These standards also reflect the ongoing process for developing and maintaining expertise within the discipline.

THE NEED TO MEASURE PROFESSIONAL DEVELOPMENT

Such standards provide a foundation for the profession. However, each speech-language pathologist has the opportunity and challenge to continue to grow beyond that foundation. Students and professionals are empowered to become the best speech-language pathologists they can be. This continued development helps enrich the individual's professional experience and enhances the perception of all speech-language pathology professionals. Continued development may also lead to distinction and recognition as an expert.

By studying the relationship between their competence level, professional development level, and treatment outcomes, clinical practitioners can self-evaluate and establish a means of **benchmarking.** Benchmarking uses measures or indicators of professional development and allows professionals to periodically evaluate development individually and in comparison to colleagues and peers. Evidence of professional growth, productivity, and clinical outcomes may have many uses, including planning professional continuing education activities that target areas for improvement or specialization. Benchmarking documents the practitioner's productivity, ability to provide services that help the client/patient achieve targeted outcomes, role within the agency or facility providing the service, as well as qualifications for employment or advancement. Agencies use individual and collective information when undergoing review by professional accrediting bodies. These data can also support recommendations for change in practice patterns.

Reliable benchmarking criteria and methods give speech-language pathologists a means of demonstrating an achieved level of expertise. Specific levels of expertise are critical to treatment efficacy; a less-capable professional would not attain comparable results. Likewise, as new information emerges in the profession, one must constantly reevaluate knowledge and skills to maintain an already achieved level of expertise.

DISTINGUISHING EXPERTS FROM NONEXPERTS

Most disciplines within the helping professions have developed standards of minimal competence and have made attempts to provide mechanisms for continued professional development. Similarly, theories and models of expertise in these disciplines have served as a mechanism for distinguishing experts from nonexperts. Although some colleagues and consumers may be better prepared than others to make this distinction, most practitioners have an intuitive ability to recognize expertise when they see it.

Although the lines of demarcation noting progress may not be clearly evident in the passage from novice to expert, it is generally agreed that this process occurs along a continuum. Such a continuum clearly recognizes differences between the preprofessional and the seasoned clinician with years of experience and specialized knowledge. Identifying the characteristics of expertise in speech-language pathology helps individuals to recognize ongoing professional development within themselves, within the discipline, and in comparison to practitioners of other helping professions.

Although the education and training process in speech-language pathology is not as extensive as that of the medical profession, the continuum of professional development is similar. The clinical fellowship experience that follows graduation with the master's degree allows essential continued professional development with professional mentoring. In addition, processes within the profession allow credentialed speech-language pathologists to earn and maintain advanced knowledge, specialized skills, and distinction among their colleagues. See Table 4.1 for a summary of these processes and awards as recognized by ASHA. Membership in and recognition by a variety of related professional associations is discussed in Chapter 6.

TABLE 4.1   Processes Through ASHA That Acknowledge Advanced Professional Development

Award/Recognition	Requirements/Qualifications
ASHA Award for Continuing Education (ACE)	Awarded when a member earns 7 ASHA Continuing Education Units (CEUs), the equivalent of 70 hours of continuing education within 36 months.
ASHA Special Interest Divisions (SIDs)	Provide opportunities and governance within ASHA; "mini-organizations within the larger framework" that develop their own missions, goals, and related activities (Lubinski & Frattali, 2001, p. 32). Allows members to focus on specific interests, network, seek related CEUs and develop policy (Kuster, 1999).
Specialty Recognition Program	Speech-language pathologists who have obtained advanced knowledge and practice experience in a particular specialty; membership is voluntary and must meet established eligibility criteria. (For examples refer to http://www.stuttering specialists.org and http://swallowingdisorders.org)
Honors of the Association	ASHA's highest award, recognizing exceptional service and distinguished contributions to the field.
ASHA Fellow	A lifetime honor that recognizes professional or scientific based contributions within and beyond one's community or state.
Distinguished Service Award	Recognizes significant contributions to the profession by nonmembers.
Dorothy Dryer Award for Volunteerism	Acknowledges extraordinary effort by members who volunteer time and other resources to ASHA.
Certificate of Recognition for Special Contributions in Higher Education	Recognizes achievement and contributions within the past five years at college and universities.
Certificate of Recognition for Special Contributions in Multicultural Affairs	Recognizes achievement and contributions by members in the areas of multicultural education, research, and clinical service.

The changing demands of service delivery in speech-language pathology accentuate the urgency of developing a description of expertise. Many pioneers of the communication disorders field achieved their expertise in a variety of other disciplines. For example, in the discipline's early days significant contributions from authorities in psychology, counseling, education, linguistics, or medicine were common. However, that expertise differs from the abilities that constitute the complex matrix of expertise unique to speech-language pathology.

Currently, with integrated skills, interests, and experiences, students in speech-language pathology are expected to rise to or exceed the required level of minimum competence to enter the field and attain ASHA's Certificate of Clinical Competence. Beyond that basic standard, individuals who achieve expertise in diagnosis and treatment of one or more of the communication disorders display traits and characteristics that others can identify, study, document, and emulate. Such characteristics, although observable, challenge the profession to devise markers to measure progress along the continuum of professional development toward expertise. The compiled abilities that constitute features of expertise in speech-language pathology (discussed in Chapter 3) include those most frequently cited.

In an early study of expertise within the discipline, Cornett and Chabon (1988) addressed the concept of expertise as an essential component of the professional attitude in clinical practice. They outlined six qualities of **professional attitude** in speech-language pathology:

1. *Expertise:* Includes the requisite knowledge and specialized skills as well as techniques often attested to by educational and certification requirements.

2. *Professional Norms:* Include codes of professional conduct and clinical accountability.

3. *Professional Identity:* Deals with issues of collegiality and professional memberships.

4. *Legal Identity:* Addresses state licensure laws that regulate professional practice.

5. *Business Acumen:* Focuses on management and financial aspects of professional practice.

6. *Personal Traits:* Relates to one's professional style (p. 49).

In addition to professional attitude, Cornett and Chabon proposed that a **scientific attitude** (representing the theoretical knowledge and scientific base) and a **therapeutic attitude** (representing interpersonal skills and caring and compassionate behaviors) were necessary to high-quality services in speech-language pathology.

In 1994, Kamhi reported limited research and knowledge "about the decision-making skills, interpersonal skills, and attitudes that characterize clinical expertise in our field" (p. 115). Additionally, Kamhi expressed concern for the lack of a theory of clinical expertise related to speech-language pathology. In 1995, Kamhi identified three categories of clinician characteristics important to providing effective therapy and represented clinical expertise:

- Knowledge base
- Procedural and problem-solving skills
- Interpersonal skills and attitudes

His study determined that novice clinicians exhibit a distinct division between the three components likely related to the degree of effort they expend to acquire the requisite knowledge base while simultaneously learning the technical aspects.

CONTINUUM OF EXPERTISE

As discussed in Chapter 3, helping professions largely agree that expertise develops in discrete stages or along a continuum (Berliner, 1991; Chi, Glaser, & Farr, 1988; Elstein, 1994; Ericsson, Krampe, & Tesch-Romer, 1993; Ericsson & Smith, 1991; Graham, 1998; Hibbard, 1995; Holyoak, 1991; Jacobs, 2003). Ball (2000) developed a model for personal and professional development (PPD) that provided a framework for a continuum of development in the art and design curriculum. This model reflects the continuum of learning from entry into the program of study through postgraduation (Table 4.2). This continuum is similar to the three-stage continuum of clinical supervision developed by Anderson (1988) to reflect the stages of support (evaluation-feedback, transitional, self-supervision) provided for graduate students in speech-language pathology.

Jacobs (2003), using a workplace perspective, distinguishes experts from others by their ability to use high levels of competence in practical ways. He describes this as the **essential nature** of expertise. As a result of this expertise, the individual consciously employs knowledge and skills to achieve outcomes of value to others. These outcomes are exemplary in comparison to those brought about by a less skilled individual. The levels of competence designated by this model include the following:

- *Novice*—One who is new to the work situation, has minimal exposure, and lacks knowledge and skills necessary to meet requirements and adequately perform.
- *Specialist*—One who can reliably perform certain components of the work unsupervised but is limited in abilities, requires coaching, and performs best in routine activities.
- *Experienced Specialist*—One who can perform specific tasks easily and with skill, is practiced, and may remain at this level for an extended time.

TABLE 4.2   Model and Framework for Personal and Professional Development

A Continuum of Learning				
Entry	$\longrightarrow$	$\longrightarrow$	$\longrightarrow$	Postgraduation
Dependence				Independence
Seeking Direction				Self-Directed
Surface Learning				Deep Learning
Focus on Product of Learning				Focus on Process of Learning
Abilities for Self-Evaluation Undeveloped				Abilities for Self-Evaluation Developing
Critical Abilities Undeveloped				Critical Abilities Developing
Unskilled				Skills Used Intuitively
Working Method Undeveloped				Working Method Used Intuitively
Student	Researcher	Investigator	Practitioner	Consultant

Adapted from Ball, L. (2000). In T. Bourner, T. Katz, & D. Watson (Eds.), *New directions in professional higher education* (p. 206). Buckingham, England: The Society for Research into Higher Education & Open University Press.

- *Expert*—One who has the knowledge and experience to meet and exceed requirements, is respected by others because of expertise, and can apply knowledge and experience to routine and novel situations.
- *Master*—One who is regarded as the expert's expert and who sets the standard of others (p. 6).

We can represent the concept of a continuum as it relates to speech-language pathology with five distinct levels of development: preprofessional, novice, competent speech-language pathologist, experienced nonexpert, and expert speech-language pathologist (see Table 4.3). Each stage may be distinguished from the others by the presence, absence, or degree of development of a variety of knowledge banks and skills inventories. The inventory for self-evaluation (Appendix A) may be used for periodic monitoring of professional development along the continuum of expertise.

Preprofessional

Students enrolled in accredited undergraduate and graduate programs of study represent the preprofessional level of development. The primary focus of activity for the preprofessional involves academic coursework and supervised practicum that prepare the student for professional practice.

Most undergraduate programs in communication sciences and disorders focus on a general educational foundation in math, science, normal speech and language

TABLE 4.3   Continuum of Expertise in Speech-Language Pathology

Level 1	Level 2	Level 3	Level 4	Level 5
Preprofessional	Novice	Competent speech-language pathologist	Experienced NonExpert	Expert

development, some introductory course work related to disorders, and observation of clinical practice. Others, however, offer limited opportunity for clinical experience.

At this level, one stumbling block to smooth passage along the professional continuum is failure to recognize early the significant impact that undergraduate academic performance can have on future opportunities for admission to graduate programs of study. Graduate programs seek to recruit qualified candidates whose academic records suggest anticipated success in advanced curriculum and who will enter the profession as a successful practitioner in one or more of a variety of contexts. Often, students fail to understand the impact of poor undergraduate performance until it is too late to reverse the situation.

Students who decide to pursue a master's (graduate) degree must soon seek information about admission criteria for targeted graduate programs. Early knowledge of admission criteria shows students what they must study and how well they must perform. Students who experience academic difficulty may benefit from the following suggestions:

- Recognize the consequences of poor academic performance (irreparable damage to the overall grade point average, dismissal from the undergraduate program, significantly reduced likelihood of admission to graduate school).
- Maintain balance in personal, social, and academic endeavors.
- Develop and use effective study habits. (Keep up with reading assignments, prepare for class in a timely manner, review early for upcoming tests, develop higher order thinking skills rather than relying on memorization, take notes in class, ask questions for clarification, seek assistance outside of class/meet with professors and instructors, focus on developing knowledge and skills not just earning the grade, and assume a professional attitude and a sense of responsibility for performance.)
- Participate in study groups.
- Utilize university and community resources for assistance in developing more effective academic strategies.
- Seek career counseling.
- Seek a professional mentor.

Graduate study involves continued clinical practice observation, lecture/discussion classes, seminars, and clinical practicum experiences. These provide information about theory, ethical conduct, methods of scientific research, biological and physical sciences, mathematics and statistics, disorder areas (articulation, fluency, voice and resonance, receptive and expressive language, hearing, swallowing, cognitive aspects of communication, social aspects of communication, and communication modalities), and supervised clinical practice in a variety of settings and across the life span.

Concurrent participation in course work and practicum allows students to develop both knowledge and skills as they apply in practice what they learn in class. Practicum also provides an opportunity to evaluate students in a context other than the classroom. Evaluation data reflect performance in clinical activities, the *what* and *how* of professional practice. Students may participate in the evaluation process through self-evaluation or rating, portfolio or reflective journal review, or assessment of client/patient clinical outcomes. Often students experience discomfort with the evaluation process because they view the process as personal and subjective. Graduate students benefit from using specific strategies to develop skills within the clinical context:

- Strive to increase independence.
- Adopt an attitude of caring and responsibility.
- Shift priorities from your needs to the needs of the client.
- Utilize time-management strategies.
- Focus on acquiring knowledge and developing skills rather than making grades.
- Take initiative in seeking assistance.

All student or preprofessional clinical practice must be supervised by an ASHA-certified professional (a current ASHA member who holds the CCC in the area of practice). In addition, the supervisor must have the appropriate state license when applicable. The amount and type of supervision must follow ASHA guidelines. Current guidelines are posted on the ASHA website in the ASHA *Certification and Membership Handbook.*

Although graduate programs offer opportunities for limited "specialization" through thesis, thesis alternatives, and other supplementary activities, the primary focus is on providing the student with a solid foundation of competence, discussed in Chapter 8, which covers knowledge and skills related to general practice of the profession. At this stage, preprofessionals begin to integrate information and skills, focus on expertise remains segmented, and factors representing expertise may develop somewhat independently.

Graduate programs in Communication Sciences and Disorders (CSD) must respond to the needs of students, accrediting bodies, clients/patients, and future employers of graduates. As a result, programs constantly monitor their curriculum's ability to meet these needs and develop improvements as trends demand. The quality of the end product—the graduate—reflects a joint effort between student and program entities (facility, curriculum, faculty, community resources that serve as off-campus placements). Education and training of future speech-language pathologists present numerous challenges to programs and to students.

These challenges are also addressed at a national level. ASHA, in 1999, identified five priority issues for the association. One of these issues specifically relates to the conflict in expectations of graduates (skills and knowledge) among academicians, practitioners, and employers. Disagreement centers on when and where students should acquire knowledge and clinical skills: in school, during the clinical fellowship (CF) year, or beyond the CF on the job. A 1997 ASHA analysis of practice patterns in speech-language pathology identified clinical activities and knowledge areas newly certified speech-language pathologists needed to perform competently. Participants in the survey included educators, practicing speech-language pathologists, supervisors of clinical fellows, and clinic directors of health-care facilities. With more than 2,800 participants responding, the results indicated the following:

- Participants strongly agreed on 53 clinical activities and 85 knowledge areas they considered important for speech-language pathologists.
- A pattern of conflicting opinion between clinical practitioners and educators indicated little agreement as to where entry-level speech-language pathologists should acquire knowledge and clinical skills.

Models for education then current apparently failed to address the differences in expectations. In response, information was disseminated about the changing workplace, the required competencies for entry-level professionals, and possible methods for programs and employers to support new professionals. The briefing paper is available on line at http://www.asha.org.

Possible solutions to challenges in educating speech-language pathologists included increased collaborative efforts, shared responsibility for educating future professionals, increased communication and partnering among all stakeholders, and more realistic expectations. In addition, students must demonstrate responsibility and must be proactive in developing their clinical skills. Also, graduate programs are challenged to emphasize critical thinking and problem-solving skills, understanding of service delivery systems (health care and educational), and helping students develop an entrepreneurial attitude toward their careers.

Novice

The novice clinician is the beginning professional. Information from the U.S. Bureau of Labor Statistics (BLS) suggests that the employment rate for speech-language pathologists is expected to grow faster than the average for other professions (out of the 700 professions monitored) through 2010. A 39 percent increase in job openings means that a total of 57,000 positions for speech-language pathologists are projected between 2000 and 2010. This need is prevalent nationwide and across practice settings, and is due primarily to growth and attrition. (See http://www.bls.gov/oco/home.htm for more specific information.)

Within the profession of speech-language pathology, the first year of practice, depending on the length of the experience, is designated as the **clinical fellowship (CF).** Clinical fellows follow ASHA guidelines in the *Certification and Membership Manual* (ASHA, 2002) for the required types of experiences and time frame as they prepare to apply for the CCC. The guidelines designate the following:

- Qualifications that include graduation from an accredited program with the appropriate distribution of coursework, passing the National Examination in Speech-Language Pathology, completion of the minimum amount of clinical experience across the life span and in the nine disorder areas in a variety of settings.
- Amount of time employed at the site and the length of the CF experience.
- Qualifications of the CF supervisor.
- Methods and schedule for evaluating the CF.
- Official reporting of the experience and the CCC application.

During the CF, the novice accepts professional responsibilities but draws on the CF supervisor for support and guidance. The novice must successfully complete the CF experience, apply for the CCC, and be able to practice independently.

While completing the CF, the novice clinician may also be fulfilling requirements for state licensure and/or teacher certification. Although some immediately enroll in doctoral programs of study to continue their education and prepare for participation in the profession in an academic context, the majority of newly certified speech-language pathologists pursue clinical practice. Novices exchange the rigor and demands of graduate study for the daily challenge of professional practice in a new setting. During this phase of professional development, the novice focuses on increasing professional contacts through networking. This informal support system includes professionals within the discipline who assist, guide, consult, and direct as necessary. Networking provides a source of aid to the novice when questions arise related to practice, policies, and conduct. This support system can also provide a context for benchmarking, an incentive for continued learning, and many valuable resources for professional development. As the novice settles into the role of practitioner, this is a time for self-evaluation relative to the five factors of expertise. Self-evaluation must be followed by intentional effort to develop plans and time lines for the future.

Entry-level clinicians in today's practice settings must successfully accomplish the following when providing clinical services:

- Navigate reimbursement systems.
- Understand the complexities of managed care.
- Understand current legislation.
- Use efficacy and outcomes data to advocate for services (http://www.asha.org).

Competent Speech-Language Pathologist

The level of competent speech-language pathologist represents a broad spectrum of practitioners providing services in a variety of settings (see the chapters in Section 3 for a discussion of practice settings). These practitioners have pursued varying degrees of professional development and have a range of years of experience. They represent the majority of speech-language pathologists and many on their way to becoming experts.

Speech-language pathologists at this stage face the following challenges:

- Take part in experimental and clinical research.
- Stay abreast of developments by reading professional publications regularly.

- Self-evaluate and formulate a plan for continuing education.
- Participate in continuing education (CE) to enhance the knowledge base and improve clinical practice.
- Consider specialization.
- Network with other professionals.
- Become active in state and national professional organizations.

In addition to meeting the day-to-day demands of practice within one or more settings, the competent clinician must act responsibly to maintain all requirements for certification, state license, and/or teacher certification as applicable. This means staying abreast of changes in rules and regulations, planning approved continuing education activities, maintaining documentation of professional training/education activities, and paying fees and membership dues in a timely manner. At this stage, professional involvement grows beyond the local level and active participation in state and national organizations is targeted. Such involvement promotes currency of knowledge of standards, guidelines, policies, and practice patterns. It also provides a means for shaping the future of the profession.

Professionals at this level make important decisions about their future careers. Decisions to change practice settings or clinical populations served may require retooling (seeking education and training that prepare the speech-language pathologist for a new area of practice). This is also the time to decide about areas for specialization and the available mechanisms for recognition as a specialist in a particular area of practice. As part of this career planning, the speech-language pathologist also makes decisions about balancing personal and professional life and how best to achieve specific goals. These decisions may affect the choice of practice setting, the amount of time and energy devoted to the professional role, the degree of involvement in professional associations, means of staying up with advances in the profession, and the amount and types of continuing education activity. The competent speech-language pathologist demonstrates independent life-long learning and professional management skills that promote success. Advancements in the knowledge base and changes in the scope of practice make this demand for continued learning and professional develop essential.

Beyond the professional knowledge base and skills inventory, ASHA identifies nine workplace success skills, targeted by competent speech-language pathologists, that graduate students need to learn (http://www.asha.org/members/phd-faculty-research/reports/changing.htm). Listed here, the skills have been keyed to the five factors of expertise presented in Chapter 3:

1. *Planning and Priority Setting*—Ability to accurately estimate task length and difficulty, formulate objectives, order task steps according to a hierarchy, make adjustments in response to arising problems, and make maximum use of resources. (Problem-Solving Skills and Technical Skills)

2. *Organization and Time Management*—Ability to coordinate several activities or tasks at once (such as goal completion, resource utilization, and documentation). (Professional Skills and Technical Skills)

3. *Managing Diversity*—Ability to appreciate and accept different personal styles, different styles of working, and cultural differences in clientele and workplace. (Interpersonal Skills)

4. *Team Building*—Ability to work within a collaborative system and within teams to share and manage clients and resources. (Professional Skills)

5. *Interpersonal Savvy and Peer Relationships*—Ability or know-how related to working with others within a setting, organization, or profession. (Interpersonal Skills)

6. *Organizational Agility*—Ability to successfully navigate organizational structures/systems and related politics. (Professional Skills and Problem-Solving Skills)

7. *Conflict Management*—Ability to negotiate common ground during conflicts, to gain the trust of others, and to demonstrate good timing. (Interpersonal Skills)

8. *Problem Solving, Perspective and Creativity*—Ability to employ innovation, objectivity, and global thinking. (Problem-Solving Skills)

9. *Dealing with Paradox and Learning on the Fly*—Ability to be flexible and to adjust one's behavior to the situation. (Problem-Solving Skills, Technical Skills, and Knowledge and Experience)

At this stage of professional development, each speech-language pathologist makes a conscious decision about a future career as a professional. Regular self-evaluation, planning, and setting professional goals encourage continued professional development. Failure to engage in these processes can result in stagnation and lack of continued development.

Experienced Nonexpert

The experienced nonexpert stage represents the professional who adheres to CCC requirements and applicable state license and or teacher certification and has many years of experience as a practitioner. Although these professionals are recognized for "staying power," they have not achieved distinction among their peers. For some, this level of development along the continuum may be a conscious decision; for others, a matter of circumstance. This career point is not necessarily negative but rather a time for caution and renewed self-evaluation and planning. Continued professional development across a career does not happen by chance. Practitioners need to follow a plan for professional development to fulfill their professional role. Although experienced nonexperts may be competent in providing services, they may not have reached their full potential as individual professionals.

Expert

The expert speech-language pathologist embodies the ideal in the profession: a standing not every professional can achieve or even desires to achieve. However, the expert serves as a resource for others, supplying the knowledge and abilities on which the reputation is founded. Expert speech-language pathologists work in a variety of settings and have earned distinction among their peers and colleagues in their primary discipline as well as those of other allied health fields and in education.

This distinction is recognized because of the expert's extraordinary performance relative to the selected features of each of the five factors of expertise:

- Interpersonal Skills
- Professional Skills
- Problem-Solving Skills
- Technical Skills
- Knowledge and Experience

By its very nature, expertise develops over time. Although even the novice has features of expertise, the true expert demonstrates consistently and consciously all factors. Chapter 3 discusses each factor and its related features.

The sum of these features, the consistent ease of application of each to the appropriate situation, the conscious knowledge, and the level of outcomes achieved in the practice of the profession set the expert apart from other practitioners. Experts often are leaders in professional organizations, and they share their expertise with others as managers, supervisors, mentors, and practitioners. They also contribute to the profession through formal and informal research. Often, experts teach others in college/university programs as full-time or adjunct faculty. We look to experts to advance the knowledge base. Experts earn recognition for the quality of services they provide to clients/patients and caregivers, for their presentations, publications, product development, and impact on legislation and regulations affecting the profession.

Experts excel beyond the typical performance of those previously identified as competent speech-language pathologists. They contribute to the profession in ways that maximize their potential for the good of their clients/patients, for their professional reputations and sense of self-satisfaction, and for the profession of speech-language pathology. They are creative in applying knowledge and techniques, and they readily recognize ways and means to improve diagnostic and treatment efforts for the benefit of the consumer, the profession and the public in a continually changing society.

SUMMARY

As speech-language pathology students move diligently through required course work and practica, they accumulate knowledge and skills that prepare them to have dramatic impact on all aspects of the discipline. Student and novice clinicians identify personal strengths, preferences, and interests that move them into the professional role of helping with a commitment to others' well-being. Experience, practice, and creative competence help developing experts acquire and refine skill and gain insights. They develop intuitive responses as each interaction introduces unique opportunities. Special talent and continuing endeavor blend person with profession to yield the qualities of expertise so essential to the growth and survival of the field.

Without its emerging experts, the future of the profession would be at risk. Access to the development of expertise is not limited. This goal lies within the reach of any speech-language pathologist through exceptional use of time, effort, ability, and opportunity. Experts of tomorrow are the preprofessionals, novices, and competent speech-language pathologists of today.

THOUGHTS FOR EXPLORATION

1. Calculate the probable number of work years in your proposed career and plot your expectations of worksite, client base, and clinical role for the first 10 years.
2. What are your strengths in the five factors of expertise within the clinical context?
3. Who are the speech-language pathologists you have observed? Where would you place them on the expertise continuum and why?
4. What are some hurdles professionals experience with each step forward in the pursuit of expertise?

REFERENCES

American Speech-Language-Hearing Association. *Certification and Membership Handbook* (2002), Speech-Language Pathology. Rockville, MD: Author.

Anderson, J. (1988). *The supervisory process in speech-language pathology and audiology.* Boston: College-Hill Publications, Little, Brown.

ASHA Supplement No. 11. (1993). Rockville, MD: American Speech-Language and Hearing Association.

ASHA Supplement No. 22. (2002). Rockville, MD: American Speech-Language and Hearing Association. http://www.asha.org

http://www.asha.org
http://www.bls.gov/oco/home.htm
http://www.bls.gov/bls/blswage.htm
http://stutteringspecialists.org
http://swallowingdisorders.org

Ball, L. (2000). In T. Bourner, T. Katz, & D. Watson (Eds.), *New directions in professional higher education*. The Society for Research into Higher Education & Open University Press.

Berliner, D. (1991). Educational psychology and pedagogical expertise: New findings and new opportunities for thinking about training. *Educational Psychologist, 26*, 145–155.

Chi, M. T. H., Glaser, R., & Farr, M. J. (1988). *The nature of expertise*. Hillsdale, NJ: Erlbaum.

Cornett, B. S., & Chabon, S. S. (1988). *The clinical practice of speech-language pathology*. Columbus, OH: Merrill.

Elstein, A. S. (1994). What goes around comes around: Return of the hypothetical-deductive strategy. *Teaching and Learning in Medicine, 6*, 121–123.

Ericsson, K. A., Krampe, R. T., & Tesch-Romer, C. (1993). The role of deliberate practice in the acquisition of expert performance. *Psychological Review, 100*, 363–406.

Ericsson, K. A., & Smith, J. (Eds.). (1991). *Toward a general theory of expertise*. Cambridge, MA: Cambridge University Press.

Graham, S. J. (1998). *Quality treatment indicators: A model for clinical expertise in speech-language pathology*. Tampa: University of South Florida.

Hibbard, S. (1995). *Two studies in expertise and clinical psychodiagnosis*. Knoxville: The University of Tennessee.

Holyoak, K. (1991). Symbolic connectivism: Toward third-generation theories of expertise. In K. Ericsson & J. Smith (Eds.), *Toward a general theory of expertise* (pp. 301–336). New York: Cambridge University Press.

Jacobs, R. L. (2003). *Structured on-the-job training: Unleashing employee expertise in the workplace*. San Francisco: Berrett-Koehler.

Kamhi, A. G. (1994). Toward a theory of clinical expertise in speech-language pathology. *Language, Speech and Hearing Services in Schools. 25*(2), 115–188.

Kamhi, A. G. (1995). Defining, developing, and maintaining clinical expertise. *Language, Speech, and Hearing Services in Schools, 26*(4), 353–356.

Kuster, J. M. (1999). Special interest division on the net. *Asha, 35*, 18.

Lubinski, R., & Frattali, C. M. (2001). *Professional issues in speech-language pathology and audiology* (2nd ed.). Canada: Singular Thomson Learning.

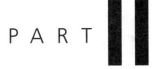

The How of Becoming an Expert

INTRODUCTION

Part II devotes five chapters to descriptions of the known characteristics of expertise in speech-language pathology. The chapters further discuss the five factors as they relate to major issues and trends within the profession. These chapters bridge the model from theory to practice.

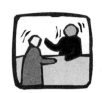

Developing Interpersonal Skills

Interpersonal Skills   Personal traits and interactive behaviors that involve both verbal and nonverbal communication between people and that influence the clinician's effectiveness.

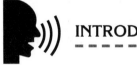

INTRODUCTION

At the heart of the therapeutic process are the clinician's *personal traits* and *interactive skills*. The conscious development and use of these traits and skills bridge the gap between being a knowledgeable, competent clinician and being a compassionate person. **Personal traits** are an individual's distinguishing characteristics that others perceive and that present a collage of "who" the person is. **Interactive skills** are essentially communicative behaviors. These characteristics and behaviors, which comprise Factor 1, Interpersonal Skills, represent an important element in developing professional expertise. In fact, expertise in interpersonal interaction depends on all of the following:

- Verbal and nonverbal communication practices of both or all participants.
- Participants' ability to perceive and comprehend intended messages.
- The professional's recognition of the relevance of the client's message to the situation.

Initial and ongoing interactive communication directly influence every treatment's success and quality.

COMMUNICATING INTENTIONALLY OR UNINTENTIONALLY

It is almost impossible not to communicate. Clinicians must constantly be aware that people communicate both verbally and nonverbally. For example, a clinician's punctuality, preparedness, and demeanor communicate volumes to the client/caregiver/family, professional colleagues, and office staff. Skilled clinicians ensure that their intended message is correctly transmitted and received (Duffy et al., 2004).

Clinical interaction, like many communications, is a two-way system that includes clinician–client, clinician–caregiver, and clinician–other professionals/staff interactions between participants (communicative partners). To ensure accurate and timely sharing of information, each partner may need to clarify or elaborate on the message, or to elicit information from the other person. Message clarification is especially necessary when one partner's (verbal and nonverbal) responses indicate misunderstanding.

INDIVIDUALITY WITHIN SPEECH-LANGUAGE PATHOLOGY

When we consider what transpires within a professional helping relationship, we look at the behaviors that show others who the helper is and the personal traits that underlie those behaviors (Karlson et al., 2004). Research in psychology and counseling has identified desirable traits of helpers: genuineness, self-disclosure, immediacy, concreteness, confrontation, empathy, congruence, warmth, and self-actualization (Speilberg, 1980).

The varied and diverse individuals who enter and have successful careers in speech-language pathology reinforce the notion that uniqueness enriches the profession. The diversity within the profession is influenced by the complexity of individual makeup. The three primary elements of individuality are covert, intermediate, and overt components. Each has important features that influence the development and expression of individuality:

- Covert components: genetic predisposition, enculturation effects such as feelings, desires, beliefs, values and principles.
- Intermediate components: organizational attributes such as valuation, judgment, assessment, and attitude; includes intention, expectation, satisfaction, acceptance, tolerance, resistance, and avoidance.
- Overt components: appearance and behavior; includes actions, inactions, and reactions.

The covert components are the basic elements of the individual's makeup. Through them the individual learns to explore the world. These core elements are derived from culture, developmental experiences, learned perceptions of self-value, and an accepted role or place in society. These elements are so deeply rooted in our lives and are so enduring that they may be hidden even from our conscious selves and at times may cause unwarranted and unexpected influences on our actions and reactions.

The intermediate components include individual traits that influence the evaluation of situations, events, ideas, persons, and their behavior. These components sustain attitude and influence reaction to people and events. They reflect intention, desire, expectations, satisfaction, tolerance, acceptance, resistance, avoidance and repulsion, which contribute to the individual's stability by modulating the external world's impact on the covert components.

The observable overt components of individuality include all the behaviors discernable through the senses. These are the physical body's actions, inactions, or reactions that enable individuals to share their ideas, feelings, and intentions. These may be consciously or unconsciously activated to influence the environment.

Certainly, communication is prominent among an individual's behaviors that others can observe. Normal communication, as well as its differences or disorders, is saturated with a significant array of covert as well as overt traits. Many factors can negatively affect communicative encounters among clients and caregivers as well as between clients and clinicians. For example, biases expressed by one or both communicating parties may create a significant stumbling block to successful communication and interaction. Such impediments must be identified and counteracted since effective communication is the primary route to positive change (Adamian, Golin, Shain, & DeVellis, 2004; Boise & White, 2004). Failure to communicate successfully results in

TABLE 5.1   Desired Traits of Speech-Language Pathologists*

Adaptable	Healthy	Tactful
	Articulate	Honest
Tolerant	Acceptance	Caring
Humble	Understanding	Active listening
Cheerful	Interested	Warm
Appropriate body language	Committed	Introspective
Well-groomed	Cultural sensitivity	Compassionate
Literate	Empathy	Concerned
Modest	Intuition	Cooperative
Nonjudgmental	Nondefensive	Courteous
Nurturing	Open-minded	Creative
Objective	Positive attitude	Dependable
Open	Reinforcing	Encouraging
Patient	Respectful	Enthusiastic
Professional	Self-motivated	Feeling
Reassuring	Sincere	Flexible
Resourceful	Trustworthy	Friendly
Sense of humor	Genuine	Sensitive
Good listener	Supportive	

*Interpersonal skills adapted from Scheuerle (1992) and additional suggestions by Graham and Guilford (2000) and Graham (1998).

misunderstanding, innuendo, gossip, and negative feelings counterproductive to clinical interactions.

PERSONAL TRAITS OF SPEECH-LANGUAGE PATHOLOGISTS

Researchers have been discussing the characteristics of individuals interested in speech-language pathology careers for many years. Scheuerle (1992) compiled an extensive list of traits considered desirable in speech-language pathologists and evident in successful clinicians. See Table 5.1. The list of traits is comprehensive.

EVALUATION OF INTERPERSONAL SKILLS

One of the greatest challenges to evaluating interpersonal skills is objectivity. Their very nature links them to self-perception, self-esteem, and self-value. Individuals who receive feedback on their interpersonal skills and on perceptions of them in a professional setting may feel defensive. To improve these skills, student clinicians and novice professionals must learn to self-evaluate and self-monitor. They must also receive feedback in a nondefensive, objective manner. The result is a broader perspective on how these skills influence effectiveness in a clinical context. Some of the desired characteristics listed in Table 5.1 (e.g., articulate, well-groomed) are readily assessed by comparing them to accepted standards. Other traits listed (e.g., introspective, humble, genuine, compassionate) are abstract and less clearly defined. Conscious evaluation of such traits and their effect within a clinical context may require focused self-study. This can be an independent self-study or one that has the help of qualified colleagues or supervisors.

SELF-STUDY

To ensure that the actions of clinicians and their influence on the client/caregiver are appropriate, sufficient, and timely, competent clinicians seek a thorough knowledge of the following:

- Self.
- How communicated messages affect observers or listeners.
- The meaning of verbal and nonverbal cues from the listener.
- Ways to assess understanding on both sides of the communication interaction (dyad).

Consequently, one essential element of professional development for novice clinicians is participation in self-study to promote self-knowledge and to foster self-awareness.

One means of self-study is to record and assess clinicians' responses to statements made by clients/patients within the clinical context. Clinician's reactions can provide insight for consciously evaluating interpersonal skills. Such an evaluation may also provide opportunities for determining possible reactions from clients/patients and implementing improved methods of responding.

Another form of self-study is to respond honestly to statements provided in clinical scenarios and evaluate the effects of those responses. The following self-study sample provides examples of this type of activity.

Self-Study Sample

Instructions: Record your spontaneous response to the following statements as if they were made directly to you by a client or caregiver.

Sample 1 A young mother states during a postclinical session conference: *I feel so guilty because my child has autism!*

   Your response: _____.

Sample 2 A client with aphasia states the following: *I've lost all of my friends since I can't play golf anymore.*

   Your response: _____.

Sample 3 A school-age child who stutters expresses the following: *I don't think that my speech is getting any better.*

   Your response: _____.

To evaluate your self-study responses, review your comments and consider the following:

- Why did you respond as you did?
- How do you *feel* about your responses?
- How do you believe the client or caregiver would *feel* about your responses?
- What *interpersonal skills* do your responses reflect?
- What desired *interpersonal skills* are absent based on your responses?
- How would you *change or modify* your responses based on your answers to the previous questions?

INTERPERSONAL COMMUNICATION AS A CLINICAL TOOL

Interpersonal communication habits—nonverbal as well as verbal—can support or detract from clinical success. Interpersonal skills are a unique and critical element of helping, and clinicians cannot risk failing to know themselves, their traits and skills, or

TABLE 5.2   Comparisons of Response Patterns Between Novice and Expert

	Novice	Expert
Approach	Courteous and respectful	Sensitive, thoughtful, and positive
Expresses	Interest and concern	Sensitivity, support, and warmth
Shares	Opinions and experience	Understanding and insight
Provides	Reassurance and information	Support

the essential equalizing behaviors essential to successful interaction with clients and caregivers from diverse social, cultural, and ethnic groups. Traits observed in novices and experts in speech-language pathology suggest that beginners are generous and attentive and that experts are involved and realistic. See Table 5.2.

Conscious observation of self and others within the clinical environment is essential for all who pursue expertise in clinical practice of speech-language pathology. By gaining **intrapersonal insight through introspection,** clinicians enhance their ability to understand the client's world by accepting the client's communication attempts without bias or judgmental reactions, thus avoiding distortion of messages across boundaries of experience, education, and ethnic or cultural background. Such openness demands flexibility as a primary ingredient of the clinician's repertoire of skills.

Students, like practitioners, must know themselves to discover the impact of the clinician's role on the clinician–client relationship. Observable conditions and actions express the clinician's attitude in ways that elicit responses from others. Novice and expert clinicians tend to exhibit varying strengths in their approach to the client's world as demonstrated by their style of interpersonal communication with clients/caregivers (Table 5.3). Those strengths arise from the knowledge, creative and novel thoughts, feelings, and experiences of the professional.

To address intimate aspects of self, each student preparing for practice in speech-language pathology must maintain an ongoing observation and assessment of personal goals, expectations, ambitions, and biases. Conscientious monitoring and realistic assessment of interpersonal skills help beginning clinicians improve their interpersonal interactions. Frequent audio and video recordings of actual clinical work are excellent opportunities to critique clinical actions and reactions. Failure to develop awareness and modify clinical behavior can inhibit or prevent future success during interactions with clients. The skilled clinician uses these insights to develop interpersonal skills that will guide the progress of treatment to achieve the client/caregiver's goals.

TABLE 5.3   A Comparison of Verbal and Nonverbal Responses in Novices and Experts

Novice	Expert
Curious	Sensitive
Inquisitive	Relevant
Friendly	Nurturing
Helpful	Knowledgeable
Developing	Experienced
Caring	Responsive
Anxious	Calm

TABLE 5.4 Selected Verbal Communicative Behaviors Proven Effective in Clinical Settings

Close-ended question	Inquiry that requires a brief, factual response
Open-ended question*	Inquiry that invites the other party to talk at length about a topic
Restatement*	The helper repeats the client's exact words, inserting second-person pronouns for *I, my,* or *me.*
Sharing	The helper reveals some aspect of personal experience relative to the client's topic.
Minimal response/ encourager	An utterance or nonverbal expression that indicates close attention and acceptance of the speaker
Silence*	Period of more than three seconds in which the helper elects to refrain from speaking
Instruction	The clinician provides new information.
Interruption	The clinician speaks while the client is talking, and the client stops talking.
Confrontation*	The clinician points out a contradiction in the client's verbal/nonverbal message.
Summarization*	The clinician reviews and presents the essence of their shared clinical experience.

(*) The asterisk identifies behaviors that experts tend to use more than do novices.

EFFECTIVE CLINICAL COMMUNICATION SKILLS

Alan Ivey and his colleagues (1971, 1997a, b) and Norman Kagan (1961) demonstrated that it is possible to identify common behaviors used in clinical interactions between the effective helper and clients/caregivers. In fact, the most readily noticeable helping skills are ordinary nonverbal and verbal communication skills typically acquired over time through social dialogue. Likewise, it is possible to identify and define potential differences between the communicating parties in a clinical setting and consequent misunderstandings in the therapeutic relationship. Resolution or compromise of such differences then becomes possible and important to the clinician–client relationship.

The practical nature of self-monitoring communicative skills or style may introduce the student to personal habitual behaviors that are natural strengths in helping. Also, students can recognize and stop other behaviors known to interfere with clinical effectiveness. Each novice clinician can independently identify usable strengths and decrease negative behaviors that hinder success. Although each communicative behavior presented in Table 5.4 can be an excellent tool, the *judicial selection and timely use* of each one now becomes the dual target of communication in clinical practice.

Accurate and timely communication between the clinician and client is critical to treatment success. For example, clinicians rely on their abilities to comprehend the information needs of clients and to supply sufficient responses (Boise & White, 2004). Too little information leaves a worrisome gap that can create client anxiety. On the other hand, too much information can overwhelm clients unready to receive or accept it and increase anxiety. The goal is to achieve open discussion of the client's concerns without the clinician reacting in a way that reflects approval or disapproval of them.

EFFECTIVE VERBAL CLINICAL COMMUNICATION SKILLS

Chermak and Scheuerle (1996) demonstrated increases in effective clinical communication skills by undergraduate students as they prepared to enter graduate school. Table 5.4 lists 10 common communication behaviors (with abbreviated definitions) specific to use in the communication disorders clinical setting. While each listed behavior is worthwhile and useful when properly applied, misuse of any one or more can deter the helping process. Five of the behaviors are marked (*) to indicate that experts tend to use these more frequently and more effectively than novices.

Discourse and dialogue style contribute to successful clinical communication. This involves knowing what to say when, the critical element of timing, as well as analyzing the listener's speech, selected vocabulary, and language comprehension level.

It can be hard to understand and modify our own habitual and casual communication practices. But we can see the need for self-awareness in the use of close-ended questions (e.g., How old are you?). In a clinical setting, overuse of closed questions can inhibit the interpersonal exchange between clinician and client or caregiver. Although such question-answer exchanges are common in initial client-interview protocols, treatment sessions that contain numerous close-ended questions can fail to elicit relevant information, produce mutual misinformation and misperceptions, or even lead to a negative client perception of the clinician.

Another communication practice to monitor and refine is the use of jargon. For example, a clinician who says "Your child received a standard score of 89 on the PPVT" may leave the caregiver wondering what he or she actually meant. Use of jargon without explanation should be limited to the professional community. Rarely does professional jargon have a place in clinical interactions with client/caregivers. When it is necessary to use jargon, the clinician must clarify or give the layperson enough information to clarify its meaning.

EFFECTIVE NONVERBAL CLINICAL COMMUNICATION SKILLS

Communication incorporates and relies on interactive characteristics and capabilities of two or more parties. The redundancy of English is helpful in clarifying messages, but the spoken language alone does not convey the speaker's full meaning. Nonverbal communication involves facial expressions and body, head, and limb movements that carry a multitude of meanings. A clinician's visible appearance and nonverbal communication often send unintended messages. We can reduce errors in communication through continuous self-examination to determine the impact of our own perceptions. That is, we must ask ourselves "What reactions do I initiate in others by my presence and behavior?" and "What reactions do the presence and actions of others initiate in me?"

Besides the nonverbal aspects of spoken language (e.g., rate, melody, rhythm, stress, loudness) certain nonverbal aspects of communication can enhance or diminish the effectiveness of a communicative effort: proxemics (space between communicators), body movements, facial expression, or influences as basic as scheduling appointments for mutual convenience. Students can approach the complex topic of nonverbal clinical communication from several points of view. The following are examples and sources of emotive information readily available to the observer:

- Body tension or movement.
- Proximity and posture.
- Facial expression that may convey information about emotion or state of well-being.
- Visual cues such as movement of hands, legs, body that require focused observation and accurate interpretation.
- Cultural differences such as those related to ethnicity, gender, sexual orientation, education level, or geographic differences and may cause a mismatch between client and clinician.

For novice clinicians, the social interactions of their childhood with parents, family, and friends, established and habituated nonverbal as well as verbal communication characteristics. They accumulated and developed through experience into a habitual communication style, which may or may not match the essential characteristics of an effective clinician.

ACQUISITION OF EFFECTIVE CLINICAL INTERPERSONAL SKILLS

The student enrolled in a speech-language pathology program may have already acquired a valuable bank of interactive behaviors but no doubt has rarely been challenged to assess and acknowledge the significance of each behavior or its potential role in clinical practice. The novice clinician who has acquired effective social communication skills and can *selectively apply* them is ready for clinical practice.

Purposeful application of interpersonal skills is critical to achieving clinical expertise in speech-language pathology. Clinicians use nonverbal and verbal behaviors in complex combinations to satisfy social communication expectations in particular settings. How clients/caregivers perceive the role of "professional" (i.e., knowledgeable authority figure in a designated environment) affects client–clinician interactions. The clinician understands the influence on that perception and uses it to further the client's therapeutic advantage. This particular part of interactive communication requires the clinician to have a thorough understanding of self and acknowledges without bias the perceptions of others.

In general, communication cannot be neutral nor without effect. That is, when people enter each others' perceptive field (i.e., seeing, hearing, or sensing another), they cannot avoid communication (Galvin & Book, 1975). Beginning clinicians may have underdeveloped interpersonal skills. Teaching interpersonal skills and clinical communication behaviors can prove difficult because they are often abstract and complex. However, learning to apply them appropriately and systematically will help a clinician become an effective instrument of change.

Based on 450 data-based studies, the work of Alan Ivey and his colleagues presents substantial evidence that interpersonal helping skills can be taught and assessed (Daniels, 2004a, b). Ordinary social interactive behaviors are easily identified, described, and enacted. Following the pattern of microteaching, it is possible to select and practice known effective interactive behaviors, one at time, so that they become a ready part of the clinician's communication behavior. In such a way, speech-language pathologists can modify habitual interpersonal actions and insert learned interactive communication behaviors proven effective in the clinical setting (Torke, Quest, Kinlaw, Eley, & Branch, 2004). As a result, clinicians gain an understanding of the power embodied in clinical communication and its influence on all individuals involved in the interaction.

 ## SUMMARY

Who you are, what you do, and how you do it affect each speech-language pathologist's level of expertise. Essential to acquiring specialized knowledge and clinical acumen are the ever-present array of personal traits and interpersonal skills. As knowledge and experience grow, speech-language pathologists develop personal insights that recognize and enhance their strengths in the area of interpersonal skills. Accurate self-understanding allows professionals to use these skills effectively in the clinical context. Self-knowledge, self-understanding, and self-acceptance benefit the treatment process and development of expertise in speech-language pathology.

 ## THOUGHTS FOR EXPLORATION

1. After observing a clinical session, identify effective interpersonal skills demonstrated by the speech-language pathologist (refer to Table 5.1).

2. Monitor the oral communication of a professional individual whom you admire. Notice particularly the facial expression, body motion, and rate of speech.
3. Rank 10 influences in your daily life from most important to least important. Then imagine and rank 10 in the daily life of your client.

REFERENCES

Adamian, M. S., Golin, C. E., Shain, L. S., & DeVellis, B. (2004). Brief motivational interviewing to improve adherence to antiretroviral therapy: Development and qualitative pilot assessment of an intervention. *AIDS Patient Care Studies, 18*(4): 229–238.

Boise, L., & White, D. (2004). The family's role in person-centered care: Practice considerations. *Journal of Psychosocial Nursing and Mental Health Service 42*(5): 12–20.

Chermak, G. D., & Scheuerle, J. (1996). Designing and teaching university courses in counseling and collaboration. *ASHA* 1996 Convention, Seattle, Washington. Unpublished.

Daniels, T. (2004a). Over 450 data-based studies provide evidence for microcounseling effectiveness. In *Microcounseling and Multicultural Development Newsletter 2004*, 2.

Daniels, T. (2004b). Personal correspondence.

Duffy, F. D., Gordon, G. H., Whelan, G., Cole-Kelly, K., Grankel, R., Buffone, N., et al. (2004). Assessing competence in communication and interpersonal skills: The Kalamazoo II report. *Academic Medicine, 79*(6): 495–507.

Galvin, K., & Book, C. (1975). *Person to person.* Skokie, IL: National Textbook Company.

Graham, S. V. (1998). Quality treatment indicators: A model for clinical expertise in speech-language pathology. Doctoral dissertation, University of South Florida, 1998.

Graham, S., & Guilford, A. (2000). Beyond competence: Development of a model of clinical expertise. American Speech-Language-Hearing Association Annual Convention, Washington, DC. Unpublished.

Ivey, A. (1971). *Microcounseling.* Springfield, IL: Charles C Thomas.

Ivey, A., Gluckstern, N. D., & Ivey, M. B. (1997a). *Attending skills* (3rd ed.). Framingham, MA: Microtraining.

Ivey, A., Gluckstern, N. D., & Ivey, M. B. (1997b). *Influencing skills* (3rd ed.). Framingham, MA: Microtraining.

Kagan, N. (1961). *Influencing human interaction.* Washington, DC: American Personnel and Guidance.

Karlson, E. W., Liang, M. H., Eaton, H., Huang, J., Fitzgerald, L., Rogers, M. P., et al. (2004). A randomized clinical trial of a psychoeducational intervention to improve outcomes in systemic lupus erythematosus. *Arthritis and Rheumatism 50*(6): 1832–1841.

Scheuerle, J. (1992). *Counseling in speech-language pathology and audiology.* New York: Macmillan.

Speilberg, G. (1980). Graduate training in helpful relationships: Helpful or harmful? *Journal of Humanistic Psychology, 20*, 57–70.

Torke, A. M., Quest, T. E., Kinlaw, K., Eley, J. W., & Branch, W. T., Jr. (2004). A workshop to teach medical students communication skills and clinical knowledge about end–of–life care. *Journal of General Internal Medicine, 10*(5, Pt. 2): 540–544.

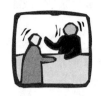

Developing Professional Skills with Membership in Professional Associations

Russell L. Malone, Frederick T. Spahr, and Arlene A. Pietranton

Professional Associations Discipline-specific organizations that develop to answer the need to structure and support educational activities; provide a formal network for interaction with others in the profession; and participate through its members in developing policies and practice parameters. Associations frequently have input on legislative issues while providing safeguards and advocacy to those whom the profession serves.

INTRODUCTION

Commitment to a professional career in speech-language pathology demands that practitioners adhere to the philosophy and principles of the national regulatory bodies that represent both public and professional expectations of its members. The professional society and its accreditation councils/committees continually confront the demands of changing times. Its national assembly and officers legislate and execute policies and programs that embody (and emphasize) profession directives, monitor the profession's progress and status as a whole, and seek equanimity among its members regardless of individual differences, preferences, or levels of expertise. Basic professional skills (Factor 2, discussed in Chapter 3) are promoted by professional associations and underlie the development of clinical expertise in speech-language pathology.

NSSCSD and AASC, Student Journal Group and Sigma Alpha Eta, Demosthenes Club, NAHSA, and IALP. The history of speech, language, and hearing associations in North America is replete with such acronyms. With few exceptions, these organizations, founded several generations ago, survive today, often with new names but similar goals. These organizations live and grow stronger, because they meet a need. They provide services and benefits, intrinsic and extrinsic to their members. Belonging to an association marks achievement and continuing growth as a professional and contributes to the journey toward expertise. Membership offers networking opportunities that further social and vocational goals such as continuing education, self-evaluation, and skills development.

Various studies have investigated the value of associations to their public. Hudson Institute (1990) analyzed 505 surveys completed by then-current or prospective members of the American Society of Association Executives. Respondents indicated the following:

- Associations enable knowledge and friendship to develop among like-minded people.
- Associations present a presence as producers/providers to potential consumers.
- Associations' central functions are not arbitrary, but evolve to enhance mutual interests.

- The public value of associations is largely a consequence of their intelligent pursuit of collective interest.
- Associations are more deeply immersed in education than in any other activity. The special value of association education is in translating research findings into concrete requirements of their discipline. This function enables associations to play a leading role in training the future workforce.
- Research programs of professional associations are central to the very mission and definition of the professions.

A 1998 study (Public Opinion Strategies, Greenberg Quinlan Research) supported the earlier finding (Hudson Institute, 1990) that member education is the most common association function. Based on responses to 274 mail questionnaires and 326 telephone interviews by chief executive officers serving as members of the American Society of Association Executives (ASAE), member education was identified as their most common association function (95%) and their single largest budget item. Seven out of 10 associations conducted industry research and three out of five set product and service standards for their services.

HISTORICAL PERSPECTIVE

Associations also have played a key role in fostering the discipline of human communication sciences and disorders. Table 6.1 highlights the development of the American Speech-Language-Hearing Association from its inception to its current status and includes major milestones for the profession.

NATIONAL SOCIETY FOR THE STUDY AND CORRECTION OF SPEECH DISORDERS

The National Society for the Study and Correction of Speech Disorders (NSSCSD), founded circa 1918, was probably the first association established for professionals in what is now the discipline of communication sciences and disorders. Public school speech correctionists

TABLE 6.1 Chronological Development of the American Speech-Language-Hearing Association and Major Milestones

1918	National Society for the Study and Correction of Speech Disorders (NSSCSD)
1925	American Academy of Speech Correction (AASC)
	—Promoted scientific and organized work in speech correction
1947	American Speech and Hearing Association (ASHA)
	—Added specialization in hearing services
1952	American Speech and Hearing Association (ASHA)
	—Established standards for the Certificate of Clinical Competence (CCC)
1958	American Speech and Hearing Association (ASHA)
	—Established the national office
	—Opened the office with two staff members
1965	American Speech and Hearing Association (ASHA)
	—established a single level of certification (master's degree)
1978 to 2006	American Speech-Language-Hearing Association (ASHA)
	—in 2004, 46 state licensure requirements included the applicant to hold the ASHA CCC
	—in 2005, the national office is staffed by 225 individuals
	—as of 2005, new standards for speech-language pathology were implemented
	—as of 2012, new standards for audiology are to be fully implemented

from the eastern states constituted most of its membership. In early 1918, NSSCSD announced the forthcoming *American Journal of Speech Disorders and Correction,* edited by society founder W. B. Swift. Although the contents page was published, the journal never materialized. Meetings of the NSSCSD reportedly continued as late as 1931 (Malone, 1999).

AMERICAN SPEECH-LANGUAGE-HEARING ASSOCIATION

The American Academy of Speech Correction (AASC) was born December 29, 1925, in the Trophy Room of New York City's McAlpine Hotel, during the 11th annual convention of the National Association of Teachers of Speech (NATS). NATS members included academicians interested in many aspects of communication. AASC stated that its purpose was the "promotion of scientific, organized work in the field of speech correction." Membership was limited to those "doing actual corrective work . . . teaching methods of correction to others, and conducting research, which has as a leading purpose the solution of speech correction problems" (AASC, 1925, p 3).

Of the 11 founding members, 2 wanted membership limited to individuals with a Ph.D.; 5 believed only the master's degree should be required. Neither "audiology" nor "hearing" was mentioned in the 1925 meeting minutes. Audiology as a profession did not exist at this time.

As the years passed, increasing numbers of members had primary interest in hearing science and disorders as an outcome of World War II. Elaine Pagel Paden, author of *History of the American Speech and Hearing Association 1925–1958* (1970) indicated that as early as 1946, the executive council recognized the need to adjust membership requirements to accommodate individuals interested in hearing disorders.

In 1947, the association recognized the presence of such professionals by changing its name from the American Speech Correction Association to the American Speech and Hearing Association (ASHA). In 1952, ASHA established two levels of certification, separate from membership—basic and advanced—with one set of requirements for specialists in speech and another for those specializing in hearing.

The association took an additional 25 years to officially recognize members' work in language by changing the practitioner title to speech-language pathologist. Two years later, the American Speech and Hearing Association became the American Speech-Language-Hearing Association. This controversial move failed when first introduced to the legislative council in 1977 but passed the following year. Although the name changed, the acronym, now familiar to influential people in government and media, remained the same, ASHA.

Today, in its 81st year, the American Speech-Language-Hearing Association is recognized as the professional, scientific, and credentialing association for more than 115,000 members and affiliates who are audiologists, speech-language pathologists, and speech, language, and hearing scientists. ASHA's mission is "to promote the interests of and provide the highest quality services for professionals in audiology, speech-language pathology, and speech hearing science, and to advocate for people with communication disabilities" (ASHA, 2005).

The founders who promoted the master's degree as the requirement for membership and those who lobbied for the Ph.D. would both be pleased today. The master's degree is currently the basic academic requirement for both professions, but as of 2012, a doctorate will be required for all new audiology certificate holders (ASHA, 2003).

The association is currently governed by a 13-person executive board and a 163-member legislative council composed of 150 voting representatives from the 50 states and the District of Columbia as well as international members, students, and the 13 executive board members. The national office opened in 1958 with a staff of two. In 2005, the staff numbers approximately 225. What accounts for this continued growth?

MEMBER SERVICES AND BENEFITS

Professional associations offer many benefits and services. The extent to which these services vary depends on the association under consideration. The following section discusses specific services of the American Speech-Language-Hearing Association, the largest provider of services for speech-language pathologists.

Certification

The association uses certification to recognize individuals, usually members, who meet its specified criteria (Malone, 1999). ASHA has been certifying professionals since 1952. The Certificate of Clinical Competence (CCC) is the most widely recognized standard of competency for speech-language pathologists and audiologists, and for many it is the first significant step toward expertise.

Many employers, including medical settings and private practices, require the ASHA CCC for employment. Various payers recognize the CCC holder as the qualified provider; employers and their clients know that the professional has met rigorous standards of competency. According to the 2005 revised standards for speech-language pathology, these standards include the following:

- Completion of a minimum of 75 semester credits culminating in a graduate degree from an ASHA-approved program in an accredited university.
- Completion of a minimum of 400 clock-hours of clinical practicum under a certified supervisor.
- Completion of 36 weeks of supervised clinical experience following receipt of the graduate degree.
- Passing a national examination (http://www.asha.org/about/membership-certification/handbooks/slp/slp_standards_new.htm.)

Certification often facilitates qualifying for a state license to practice within the 46 states that as of November 2004 require licensing for speech-language pathologists.

ASHA certification is recognized as the model of competence within the professions and by those in health-care and education fields. Qualifying for the CCC demonstrates the holder's commitment to excellence.

Continuing Professional Development

The master's and/or doctoral degrees demonstrate that the holder has mastered a critical body of material, an important educational stage for audiologists and speech-language pathologists. The CCC attests to the speech-language pathologist's clinical knowledge. But because the speech-language pathologist seeking expertise will not settle for minimal competencies, the expert speech-language pathologist is always a work in progress. As research continues to create new knowledge, speech-language pathologists and audiologists refine clinical skills by assessing research findings and applying them appropriately in clinical contexts.

Opportunities for professional development and continuing education are major benefits of belonging to a professional association that offers publications, conventions, and workshops. Many associations and licensing boards require demonstration of continued professional development for maintaining credentials.

Publications

ASHA publishes five periodicals and e-mail newsletters. The *Journal of Speech, Language, and Hearing Research* (*JSLHR*) is produced five times a year. *JSLHR* is the premier research journal of the speech-language pathology and audiology professions. It includes articles relating to the processes and disorders of hearing, language, and speech, including their diagnoses and treatment.

Language, Speech, and Hearing Services in Schools (*LSHSS*) is one of the more valuable journals for the approximately 55% of members who work in educational settings. Published quarterly, *LSHSS* presents up-to-date information on all aspects of clinical speech, language, and hearing services to children and adolescents, particularly in school settings.

The *American Journal of Speech-Language Pathology: A Journal of Clinical Practice* is published quarterly. It addresses all aspects of clinical practice in speech-language pathology, including screening, assessment, and treatment techniques; prevention; professional issues; supervision; and administration.

The *American Journal of Audiology: A Journal of Clinical Practice* (*AJA*) is published semiannually. *AJA* addresses all aspects of clinical practice in audiology, including screening, assessment, and treatment techniques; prevention; professional issues; supervision; and administration.

The ASHA Leader is a four-color publication printed 16 times a year as of 2005. Contents include in-depth features, news articles, classifieds, and letters to the editor related to the professions. Supplements are published periodically.

E-mail newsletters include *Access Schools, Access SLP Health Care,* and *ASHA Headlines.* All are available by sending a blank e-mail from your own account. *Access Schools* addresses specific needs of school-based speech-language pathologists and is available as a bimonthly update during the school year (http://www.asha.org). *Access SLP Health Care* is a bimonthly e-newsletter that addresses the specific needs of speech-language pathologists working in health care (http://www.asha.org). *ASHA Headlines* provides updates on government relations, public relations, audiology, and SLP practices issues and activities as well as executive director updates and periodic summaries of various ASHA committee, board, and council meetings (http://www.asha.org).

ASHA members receive the *ASHA Leader,* their choice of one other journal, and access to all journals online as part of their membership dues. Members may also subscribe to the other journals at reduced rates. Membership in other professional associations provides additional journals, websites, and electronic mailings that may be useful in gaining expertise and remaining current in one's practice. A list of other related associations is provided at the end of this chapter.

Convention and Workshops

ASHA offers programs designed to give practitioners tools to improve their clinical decision making: updated clinical and research information, examples of best practices, and models of effective delivery service. In 2005, thousands of members traveled to San Diego to take advantage of more than 1,500 opportunities to expand their knowledge at ASHA's 80th annual convention. They chose from short courses, computer labs, and technical sessions.

ASHA routinely offers its members many continuing-education opportunities. These include live in-person conferences, telephone seminars, live and self-study Web workshops, multimedia self-study programs, and print-based self-studies, accessible online or in print.

Special Interest Divisions

Sixteen special interest divisions allow ASHA members and students to participate in a range of special interest areas, including fluency, language, voice, speech science, swallowing, gerontology, culturally and linguistically diverse populations, and augmentative communication. Membership in special interest divisions and working with peers who have specialized experience in a specific area is an additional way to gain expertise.

Website

ASHA maintains and continually updates a state-of-the-art website (http://www.asha.org). Members can access hundreds of thousands of pages on a wide range of professional topics 24 hours a day, 7 days a week. Member forums provide online networking among members.

Award for Continuing Education (ACE)

The ACE is the formal recognition of professionals who have demonstrated their commitment to lifelong learning by earning a specified number of continuing education units (CEUs) within three years.

ASHA CE Registry

The registry uses a computerized database to help CCC holders (members and non-members) track their CEUs in a permanent, cumulative transcript. In addition, the registry helps individuals to locate continuing education opportunities.

Advocacy

ASHA's national office supports its mission "to promote the interests of and provide the highest quality services for professionals in audiology, speech-language pathology, and speech and hearing science, and to advocate for people with communication disabilities" (ASHA Mission Statement online at http://www.asha.org) by employing lobbyists and public relations practitioners. They work with members, professional staff, state associations, and key organizations to shape and promote the messages delivered to government officials and the general public.

Code of Ethics

One of the earliest concerns of ASHA's founders was to establish guidelines for the professional conduct of members. At their initial 1925 meeting, one of the two principle reasons given for founding the association was "to establish scientific standards and codes of ethics" (American Academy of Speech Correction, 1925). The second principle reason was to encourage others to join the professions.

In 1930, the academy amended its constitution to specify behavior considered inappropriate and grounds to bar a candidate from association membership. Through the years, ASHA's code of ethics has been modified many times, most recently in 2003. Generally speaking, experts are most often knowledgeable about their code of ethics and scope of practice as these are essential for professional development and practice. Today, the code consists of four principles as seen in Table 6.2.

TABLE 6.2 Basic Principles of the ASHA Code of Ethics (2003)

Individuals shall honor their responsibility to hold paramount the welfare of persons they serve professionally or participants in research and scholarly activities and shall treat animals involved in research in a humane manner.

Individuals shall honor their responsibility to achieve and maintain the highest level of professional competence.

Individuals shall honor their responsibility to the public by promoting public understanding of the professions, by supporting the development of services designed to fulfill the unmet needs of the public, and by providing accurate information in all communications involving any aspect of the professions, including dissemination of research findings and scholarly activities.

Individuals shall honor their responsibilities to the professions and their relationships with colleagues, students, and members of allied professions. Individuals shall uphold the dignity and autonomy of the professions, maintain harmonious inter-professional and intra-professional relationships, and accept the professions' self-imposed standards.

Employment

The *ASHA Leader* publishes a classified section in each issue. In addition, the annual convention provides opportunities to meet with potential employers. ASHA and its student affiliate, the National Student Speech Language Hearing Association, offer a variety of materials to guide the job seeker. In addition, ASHA provides an online career center at http://www.asha.org/about/career/.

THE NATIONAL STUDENT SPEECH LANGUAGE HEARING ASSOCIATION

The National Student Speech Language Hearing Association (NSSLHA) is the pre-professional membership association for part- or full-time students interested in the study of communication sciences and disorders.

NSSLHA is the offspring of a merger that followed 12 years of interaction between Sigma Alpha Eta and the ASHA Student Journal Group. Sigma Alpha Eta was founded by Eugene McDonald at The Pennsylvania State University in 1946. Charlotte Brong, Louisiana State University, served as executive director from 1949 to 1960. ASHA proposed an affiliation with Sigma Alpha Eta in the early 1960s. When the students rejected ASHA's proposal in 1965, ASHA formed the Student Journal Group.

Five years later, Sigma Alpha Eta reopened discussions, but this time ASHA hesitated. In 1972, after two years of negotiations, Sigma Alpha Eta merged with the ASHA Journal Group to create the National Student Speech Language Hearing Association. In 2004, NSSLHA had approximately 11,000 members with chapters in more than 301 colleges and universities. Benefits of NSSLHA membership may be seen in Table 6.3. Further information concerning NSSLHA is at the NSSLHA website (http://www.NSSLHA.org).

TABLE 6.3   Benefits of National Student Speech Language Hearing Association Membership

Personal and Professional Aspects of Membership	Recognition among colleagues and professionals of interest in the study of communication and its disorders.
	Networking with others with similar professional interests leading to social and employment opportunities.
Publications	Receipt of:
	Contemporary Issues in Communication Science and Disorders (CICSD), a NSSLHA publication
	News and Notes, NSSLHA's newsletter *ASHA Leader*, ASHA's news publication
	A choice of one of the following ASHA journals:
	American Journal of Audiology (AJA)
	American Journal of Speech-Language Pathology (AJSLP)
	Journal of Speech, Language, and Hearing Research (JSLHR)
	Language, Speech, and Hearing Services in Schools (LSHSS)
	Access to "members only" areas of the ASHA and NSSLHA websites
Financial Advantages	Reduced registration fee for ASHA Convention
	Discounted membership in ASHA's special interest divisions
	Discounts on ASHA and NSSLHA products
	Discount on dues for first year of ASHA membership and certification

AMERICAN SPEECH-LANGUAGE-HEARING FOUNDATION

The American Speech-Language-Hearing Foundation was founded in Iowa City in 1939 as the Demosthenes Club, named after the famous Greek whose path to fame as an orator is alleged to have been precipitated by his stuttering. Its purpose, recorded by founder Wendell Johnson, "grew out of efforts made by speech defectives [sic] themselves to stimulate the development of speech correction in the United States" (Malone, 1999, p. 193). (Incidentally, Dr. Wendell Johnson served as chair of the foundation from 1946 to 1960 and was ASHA president in 1950.) Chapters were formed in some states and as far away as Johannesburg, South Africa. In 1946, ASHA's executive council incorporated the club, by then known as the Speech Correction Research Foundation, as a unit of the American Speech Correction Association, ASHA's name from 1934 to 1947.

Forty-eight years later, in 1994, the Speech Correction Research Foundation, now known as the American Speech-Language-Hearing Foundation (ASHF), separated from ASHA. Today, the foundation remains true to its founding goals of promoting better quality of life for children and adults with communication disorders. Its mission is to advance knowledge about the causes and treatment of hearing, speech, and language problems.

To achieve its goals, the foundation raises funds from individuals, corporations, and organizations in support of research grants, graduate education scholarships, and the funding of special projects that foster discovery and innovation in the discipline of communication sciences and disorders.

NATIONAL ASSOCIATION FOR HEARING AND SPEECH ACTION

The National Association for Hearing and Speech Action (NAHSA) has, throughout its more than 80 years, consistently worked to educate the public about the needs of persons with communication disorders. NAHSA introduced Better Hearing Week in 1927.

Hearing Week became a national event in 1937 when First Lady Eleanor Roosevelt promoted it through her daily newspaper column and on her syndicated radio show. Mrs. Roosevelt's son, James, reported that she appreciated her hearing aid because of the many functions she attended. However, she would frequently turn her hearing aid off when she became weary of listening to a speaker. National Hearing Week extended to a month in May 1958, and four years later, when the association expanded its goals, it was renamed Better Hearing and Speech Month.

Troubled with repeated financial problems, NAHSA fended off demise with a grant from the Vocational Rehabilitation Administration in the 1960s. The association survived in the 1970s when a benefactor bequeathed the organization $75,000. In 1979, however, having exhausted its finances and its hopes, NAHSA became the consumer affiliate of the American Speech-Language-Hearing Association.

Today, NAHSA continues to promote public awareness of and education about communicative disabilities, the help available, and the need for early intervention. NAHSA publishes and distributes more than two dozen booklets and brochures and offers a toll-free telephone number for consumer information (800-638-8255). For 20 years, ending in 2002, NAHSA and ASHA cosponsored the Communication Awards. These awards were a project of the National Council on Communication Disorders, founded in 1979 by Kenneth O. Johnson. During its existence, the achievements of more than 200 individuals and 45 groups were recognized at various sites including the Kennedy Center, French Embassy, and ASHA Conventions.

STATE SPEECH-LANGUAGE-HEARING ASSOCIATIONS

Every state as well as the District of Columbia has a speech-language-hearing association. In many ways, state associations duplicate the work ASHA does on a national level. They actively sponsor continuing education activities and advocate for the professions and consumers, particularly with state legislatures and state regulatory agencies, including licensing boards. ASHA maintains a close relationship with these associations and assists their efforts through analysis of proposed legislation, development of model legislation, information on trends in other states, consultation on strategy, and written and oral testimony. State associations have made important achievements in the area of state licensing and client caseloads.

The Florida Speech-Language-Hearing Association (FLASHA) is a notable example of what state associations have achieved. In 1969, working against strong opposition and with little support, FLASHA members achieved the nation's first state licensing for speech-language pathologists and audiologists.

More recent achievements have been in the area of salary. Many states provide teachers who hold a master teacher certificate from the National Board for Professional Teaching Standards (NBTS) with a substantial salary supplement. Although no category is specific to speech-language pathologists or audiologists, both groups may pursue NBTS recognition. The Mississippi Speech-Language-Hearing Association convinced their state legislature that school speech-language pathologists and audiologists who hold the Certificate of Clinical Competence met standards at least as stringent as those of the NBTS. Following several years of continuous and intense dialogue with Mississippi legislators, MSHA succeeded. In 1999, legislation passed providing Mississippi school speech-language pathologists and audiologists with an annual $6,000 supplement.

Following MSHA's success, the Delaware, Missouri, and Oklahoma state associations obtained salary supplements for their school professionals in 2004. Louisiana (2003) and Oklahoma (2004) state legislatures approved the concept, but they must still allocate the money to implement the law.

State associations have been successful in passing health-related legislation. In 1998, only 11 states required that newborn babies receive a hearing screening before being discharged from the hospital. Today, 42 states and the District of Columbia have early hearing detection and intervention laws that apply to all babies. Assisted by model legislation developed by ASHA, state speech-language-hearing associations spurred this growth by joining in coalition with other professional and consumer groups to support passage of the legislation.

INTERNATIONAL ASSOCIATIONS

Founded in 1924, The International Association of Logopedics and Phoniatrics (IALP) is housed in the Netherlands (http://www.ialp.info). This organization of 56 affiliated national societies from 38 countries represents more than 130,000 members. In addition, it has individual members from 54 countries. Applicants for individual membership must be recommended by two current IALP members and professionally educated and trained within the field of communication disorders and sciences. The association's mission is to help persons with communication and swallowing disorders.

IALP publishes *Folio Phoniatrica* six times a year, in three languages, covering a broad range of international research. IALP will hold its triannual congress in Copenhagen in 2007 (http://www.ialp.info).

With its official seat in Geneva, the International Society of Audiology (ISA) states that it includes

> the science of hearing, the modeling of the auditory system, the management of hearing impaired people, both of the very young with their special problems of language development and of the elderly with the social implications of hearing impairment for work and social integration (http://www.isa.org).

Full membership in ISA requires a degree in audiology or a related field and work in the field of audiology. Student membership is available.

ISA publishes the *International Journal of Audiology,* a newsletter, in cooperation with regional and national societies, and holds a biannual congress.

QUADRILATERAL MUTUAL RECOGNITION AGREEMENT

The Quadrilateral Mutual Recognition Agreement, a recent multinational initiative, went into effect January 1, 2005. Parties to the agreement are ASHA, the Canadian Association of Speech-Language Pathologists (CASLPA), the Royal College of Speech and Language Therapists (Great Britain), and the Speech Pathology Association of Australia, Limited. This agreement in part frees members of CASLPA, the Royal College, and Speech Pathology Australia from having their course work and clinical practicum evaluated when they apply for ASHA certification. Royal College and Speech Pathology Australia members must take the Praxis exam; CASLPA members need not. CASLPA and Speech Pathology Australia must complete the clinical fellowship—36 weeks of supervised clinical practice following graduation—or equivalent. ASHA-certified members who desire certification from the Canadian, British, and Australian associations must also meet certain requirements. CASLPA requires documented evidence of prescribed clinical practicum hours and university transcripts. Speech Pathology Australia and the Royal College require the clinical fellowship year or 1,000 hours of practice completed within the past five years. Speech Pathology Australia also requires that individuals certified by ASHA before 1998 demonstrate competency in the area of dysphagia. The Royal College grants certification for one year only. Certification beyond that year requires evidence that the practitioner satisfactorily completed a year of monitored practice in the United Kingdom.

OTHER PROFESSIONAL AND SPECIAL INTEREST ORGANIZATIONS

Various organizations have evolved to serve the interests of speech-language pathology and audiology. Some of these are

➤ Academy of Dispensing Audiologists
www.audiologist.org

➤ Academy of Rehabilitative Audiology
www.audrehab.org

➤ Academy of Neurologic Communication Disorders and Sciences
www.ancds.org

➤ American Academy of Audiology
www.audiology.org

➤ American Cleft-Palate-Craniofacial Association
www.cleftline.org

- ➤ Audiology Foundation
  www.audfound.org

- ➤ American Psychological Association
  www.apa.org

- ➤ Communication Disorders Prevention and Epidemiology Study Group
  www.shrs.pitt.edu/superlectures.htm/ or
  www.omni.ac.uk/mesh/d003147.htm/

- ➤ Council for Exceptional Children
  www.cec.sped.org

- ➤ Council of Graduate Programs in Communication Sciences and Disorders
  www.capcsd.org

- ➤ Council of School Supervisors
  www.csa-nyc.org

- ➤ Council of Supervisors in Speech-Language Pathology and Audiology
  www.asha.org [new window]

- ➤ Early Childhood Education
  www.PennFoster.edu

Multicultural Constituency Groups:

- ➤ Asian-Indian Caucus
  www.asha.org/about/leadership-projects/multicultural/

- ➤ Asian Pacific Islander Caucus
  www.apiuu.org

- ➤ Hispanic Caucus
  www.chci.org

- ➤ Lesbian, Gay, Bisexual and Transgendered Audiologists and Speech-Language
  Pathologists (L'GASP)
  www.uschsc.edu/glbt/professional_organizations.htm

- ➤ National Black Association for Speech-Language and Hearing (NBASLH)
  www.nbaslh.org

- ➤ Native American Caucus
  www.nativeamericancaucus.com

You will find more information about each of the groups mentioned in this chapter at their websites or by calling ASHA's Action Center (1-800-498-2071). Participation in these types of associations and interest groups exposes professionals aiming to develop expertise in a specialized area to advanced learning opportunities. Participation will certainly help reach that goal.

SUMMARY

Students of speech-language pathology are fortunate that those who came before them did the work necessary to establish a strong, dynamic, respected, and independent profession. Speech-language pathology today is the result of dedicated and skilled professionals—educators, clinicians, and researchers—working independently at their profession and together in their associations to ensure that children and adults with communication disorders receive the quality of service they require. Pre-professionals who complete a program of study develop a solid foundation upon which to build. As professionals become certified and assume leadership roles in local, state and national associations, they continue along the journey to becoming an expert. Students initiate the journey toward expertise by becoming active in the National Student Speech-Language-Hearing Association. Throughout their professional life, they should look for opportunities through professional associations that will enhance their knowledge and skills. Additional progress toward becoming an expert may also come through membership in special interest divisions, state, and other associations.

THOUGHTS FOR EXPLORATION

1. What are five ways in which a novice clinician can effectively participate in professional association(s) of speech-language pathology?
2. How can participating in an association provide you with opportunities for professional growth and development?
3. What activities can professionals take part in to advocate for the people they serve?

REFERENCES

American Academy of Speech Correction. (December 1925). Unpublished minutes, 3.

Association Services. (1998). Washington, DC: Public Opinion Strategies & Greenberg Quinlan Research.

American Speech-Language-Hearing Association. (http://www.asha.org, 2005).

American Speech-Language-Hearing Association. (2003). Code of ethics (revised). *ASHA Supplement, 23*, 13–15.

American Society of Association Executives. (1990). *Hudson Institute Report*. Bethesda: Author.

International Association of Logopedics and Phoniatrics, (www.ialp.info, 2005).

Malone, R. (1999). *The First 75 Years*. Rockville, MD: American Speech-Language-Hearing Association.

National Student Speech-Language-Hearing Association. At http://NSSLHA.org, 2004.

Paden, E P. (1970). *History of the American Speech and Hearing Association 1925–1958*. Rockville, MD: American Speech-Language-Hearing Association.

CHAPTER 7

Problem Solving and Treatment Integrity

Jacqueline J. Hinckley

> **Evidence-Based Practice (EBP)**   A systematic method that provides scientific evidence for effective treatment of a given disorder. EBP enables clinicians to select an appropriate treatment based on a reasonable expectation of benefit.

INTRODUCTION

The evolution and perpetuation of speech-language pathology depends on the contributions of each generation of practitioners. Students who study the required educational curricula gain experience in reading, analyzing, and using research publications to identify and solve problems related to discipline content and develop many approaches to creative problem solving. The natural product of creative problem solving (e.g., problem identification, analysis, and solution) is gathered evidence that supports one treatment's effectiveness over others' under specific circumstances and in certain conditions. The importance of problem-solving skills (Factor 3 of clinical expertise discussed in Chapter 3) encompasses valuing and contributing new knowledge to the discipline for the benefit of clients and the status of the profession as a whole.

The practicing clinician faces almost daily challenging opportunities in which to develop various clinical and professional skills. Over years of practice, the hundreds of exemplars of various clinical challenges begin to generalize into typical patterns of decision making. Thanks, however, to human individuality and variability, an experienced clinician can find a challenge in the next client who walks through the door.

Take, for example, the case of a new client whose language profile is consistent with a Broca's-type aphasia (predominantly expressive aphasia). A clinical aphasiologist with several years of experience knows well-documented treatment techniques for agrammatic aphasia. In addition, the clinician most likely has experience using these techniques and understands the published scientific basis for treatment of agrammatic aphasia. This combination of experience and knowledge will likely steer the clinician toward a particular treatment approach.

Imagine further that the client also has visual agnosia. The most familiar treatment procedures for agrammatic aphasia all somewhat depend on visual stimuli. How can the clinician expand the repertoire of familiar treatments for agrammatic aphasia to accommodate this client's particular set of characteristics and circumstances? Is there one treatment not reliant on visual stimuli that would be appropriate for this client? Can the visually dependent treatment be adapted and administered in a nonvisual way for this particular client? If the treatment procedure is adapted and modified in some way, how might that affect the outcomes normally expected from this unmodified treatment?

Does adjusting the treatment detract from its potency? Might administering the altered treatment waste everyone's time and money?

Every clinician faces comparable questions and challenges and manages them in the best way possible under the immediate circumstances. Clinicians may hear a colleague say, "Well, I did this particular treatment because I just wasn't sure what to do. I've never had to handle this combination of circumstances before." Challenging combinations of circumstances call on the expert clinician to use problem-solving skills developed and tested over years of experience.

SELECTING TREATMENT OPTIONS

This chapter discusses issues related to selecting and administering treatments in an expert way. An expert has to know the treatment options available under a particular set of circumstances, weigh the potential benefits and risks of each, consider his or her qualifications to administer the most appropriate treatment, and do so with reasonable expectation of benefit. The American Speech-Language-Hearing Association Code of Ethics (ASHA, 2003) provides standards for these practices as described in Chapters 6 and 8. Evidence-based practice provides a systematic approach to considering treatment options and expected benefits for a particular client. Understanding treatment integrity in research and its implications for clinical practice contribute to decisions about how to administer any selected treatment. Finally, the expert clinician assimilates this scientific knowledge with clinical experience and integrity to generate the best possible course of action for a client.

EVIDENCE-BASED PRACTICE: BASIC STEPS

The ASHA Code of Ethics (ASHA, 2003), Principle I, Rule G, states that services should only be rendered "when benefit can reasonably be expected." Expectation of benefit can arise from two sources: scientific evidence and clinical experience. In this section we consider the principles of evidence-based practice (EBP), and how they should be incorporated into an ethical, expert practice.

Simple contact between a qualified clinician and a client is not sufficient to produce benefit. The well-documented placebo effect is typically used as a control against which to measure a treatment's potential effects. Unfocused contact in a clinical environment is a neutral position against which we deem "benefit" as improvement beyond the neutral, placebo condition.

Given a client's profile, selecting an inappropriate treatment is unacceptable. It is well documented that selecting a treatment not matched to the client's needs can produce no benefit, or possibly, deterioration. For example, a mismatch between the level of a lexical deficit in aphasia and the corresponding type of treatment, semantically or phonologically based, can produce a poorer outcome (Drew & Thompson, 1999).

Fortunately, EBP provides systematic techniques with which we can weigh the scientific evidence for treatment of a given disorder and helps the expert clinician select an appropriate treatment with reasonable expectation of benefit. EBP is the integration of "individual clinical expertise with the best available external clinical evidence from systematic research" (Sackett, Rosenberg, Gray, Haynes, & Richardson, 1996, p. 711; also cited in ASHA, 2004b). EBP derives from the observation that expert opinion alone is insufficient for appropriate clinical decision making, and could produce deleterious results. ASHA's recent technical report on EBP (2004a, b, c) provided an overview of EBP's principles and procedures, described the importance of EBP to speech-language pathology and audiology, raised awareness of EBP in the professions, and recommended ways to incorporate principles of EBP in the research base of communication disorders (ASHA, 2004b). Three important steps for implementing EBP are:

- Ask an answerable clinical question
- Identify the available evidence to address the question.
- Evaluate the evidence for its validity, impact, and applicability.

Develop Answerable Questions

The first step toward using EBP principles as clinicians is to develop questions answerable by seeking out applicable research. Appropriate clinical questions for an EBP approach should include a specified client characteristic or clinical disorder, both the intervention in question and a comparison intervention (or no intervention), and a desirable outcome important to the client (Sackett, Straus, Richardson, Rosenberg, & Haynes, 2000). For example, a clinician might ask, "Is fluency treatment more effective than no treatment for five-year-old children who stutter?"

Identifying Evidence

The second step in incorporating EBP into an ethical, expert practice is to locate scientific evidence that evaluates treatment of a particular disorder. Thus, expert clinicians must continuously monitor the developing research in their typical areas of practice. This can be accomplished by regularly attending workshops and conferences that offer scientific updates on treatment techniques. Monitoring ASHA journals and publications, including online resources, is another important way to keep abreast of scientific advances in treatment. Additionally, periodic searches of particular scientific resources, easily accomplished online, also help expert clinicians maintain contact with the scientific treatment literature.

Pursuing current techniques exposes the clinician to a range of scientific evidence. But following single studies as they are published is different from knowing the weight of all evidence in a particular practice area taken together. An important tenet of EBP is to weigh the evidence and consider the type of evidence available for any given treatment. If a new treatment sounds "just right" for a challenging client, is one study a reasonable evidence base for expectations of benefit?

One way to weigh the evidence is to consider the type of evidence provided by a particular research study. ASHA has characterized different types of experimental studies in four levels of evidence (Robey, 2004) adapted from the Scottish Intercollegiate Guideline Network. These levels of evidence are listed in Table 7.1. The levels of evidence prioritize sources of scientific evidence for treatment or other clinical procedures. The randomized controlled trial figures prominently in this ranking. An experiment in which participants are randomly assigned to treatment or control conditions provides a statistical basis for taking into account individual variability. The control condition in such a study creates a baseline or placebo against which to measure the treatment's potential effect.

When enough of these randomized controlled trial studies have been completed for a particular treatment or disorder area, it is possible to conduct a meta-analysis of the studies. A **meta-analysis** statistically analyzes the results of several studies (Robey &

TABLE 7.1   Levels of Evidence According to ASHA's Technical Report on Evidence-Based Practice

Level Ia:	Well-designed meta-analysis of >1 randomized controlled trial
Level Ib:	Well-designed, randomized controlled study
Level IIa:	Well-designed controlled study without randomization
Level IIb:	Well-designed quasi-experimental study
Level III:	Well-designed nonexperimental studies, that is, correlational and case studies
Level IV:	Expert committee report, consensus conference, clinical experience of respected authorities (ASHA, 2004)

Dalebout, 1998). The result demonstrates the weight of the evidence across several studies supporting or refuting a particular treatment's effectiveness.

Among the lower levels of evidence that do not include randomization are single-subject designs, and correlational and case studies. The weakest form of evidence is the clinical experience of respected authorities in a given specialization.

Evaluate the Evidence

One consideration for evaluating the evidence, then, is to determine what type of evidence is available for a particular intervention or technique by assessing the levels of evidence across the studies pertaining to the question. But the expert clinician will be less than satisfied with a simple count of randomized or single-subject studies available for any particular question. It is important to compare the outcomes of a particular intervention or technique across multiple studies, even ones that use different measures. What does it mean for clinical practice if one study reports an improvement of an intervention on one test or measure, and another study with a similar design reports improvement on a different measure? How can a clinician compare outcomes across different metrics?

One technique for comparing outcomes across studies is to report and evaluate effect sizes. **Effect sizes** are a family of indices that reflect on the magnitude of a treatment effect, and therefore add information to simple reporting of a statistical difference (Cohen, 1988). Most treatment studies compare the mean performances of groups or of participants in conditions (treatment or no treatment, or the comparison of two treatments) by applying a statistical test such as a **t-test** or an **F-test** (e.g., **ANOVA**). A statistically significant difference between the groups rejects the null hypothesis that the two groups performed equally. It suggests that the performance difference between the two groups is not by chance. One way to calculate an effect size is to compare the two group means in relation to their variability as measured by the standard deviation, without respect to sample size. This value is interpreted as reflecting how important the difference between the two groups may be. Cohen suggested general guidelines for interpreting this common effect size (known as **Cohen's d**). When $d = 0.2$, the effect is considered small, a medium effect is generally interpreted when $d = 0.5$, and a large effect can be associated with $d = 0.8$.

Another way to think about effect sizes is by estimating the percentage of overlap between a treatment group and a nontreatment group. Complete overlap between the two groups (no performance difference between groups) is related to an effect size of 0.0, whereas nearly complete nonoverlap between the two groups would be associated with an effect size of 2.0.

A clinician who wants to evaluate the strength of evidence for a particular treatment can use ASHA's levels of evidence (Robey, 2004) to evaluate the research designs used in the published literature. Meta-analyses, if available, can be important in weighing the evidence across studies. Finally, effect sizes either reported in the published studies themselves, or calculated by the active research consumer can shed light on the importance of a particular treatment result.

EVIDENCE-BASED PRACTICE: PRACTICE GUIDELINES

As the evidence for a treatment of a particular disorder accumulates, researchers derive classes of treatments and develop an established set of terms to reflect the degree of evidence for a particular clinical practice. **Standards** are accepted principles of patient care based on a high degree of certainty and Level I or strong Level II evidence (see Table 7.1). **Guidelines** reflect a moderate degree of certainty, are neither fixed protocols nor rigid treatment rules, and are typically based on Level II evidence. **Options** are possible treatment strategies based on limited certainty or conflicting evidence or opinion.

The Academy of Neurologic Communication Disorders and Sciences (ANCDS) is undertaking a coordinated effort to develop practice guidelines for treatment of neurogenic disorders based on scientific evidence. ANCDS seeks to develop practice guidelines for each major area of neurologic communication disorders, including acquired apraxia of speech, dysarthria, aphasia, cognitive-communicative impairment, and dementia. Golper (2001) describes practice guidelines as "explicit descriptions of how patients should be evaluated and treated," designed to "improve and assure the quality of care by reducing unacceptable variation in its provision" (p. x). The ANCDS project to develop evidence-based practice guidelines entails systematic and exhaustive literature reviews evaluated against established criteria. These reviews produce published findings that summarize the weight of published evidence for any particular treatment or assessment for use by clinicians (Frattali, Bayles, Beeson, Kennedy, Wambaugh, & Yorkston, 2003).

As practice guidelines in all areas of speech-language pathology are developed, the clinician will be able to rely on compiled evidence in support of particular treatments or disorders. The clinician should be familiar with sources that compile treatment evidence in the typical area of practice and use that evidence for making treatment decisions. Appendix B lists resources for finding summaries of evidence on treatment.

ASHA (2004a, b, c) has published recommended guidelines for the decision-making process when incorporating a treatment technique into practice, and these are reprinted in Table 7.2. The decision-making questions break down into broad steps. First, the clinician should understand the treatment, including who and under what circumstances it is recommended, and what the typical outcomes are. The clinician should know what clinical experience or training is recommended before using the treatment. It is important to assess whether the treatment fits into both the speech-language pathology professional scope of practice and one's personal scope of practice.

The second category of questions pertains to informing oneself about external sources that help to evaluate the treatment and its usefulness. Consult the ASHA website and Desk Reference to locate position statements, technical reports, or reports on competencies that pertain to the treatment or practice area. Then, search other scientific sources to determine the level and weight of evidence available to support the treatment's use and effectiveness. Finally, consulting others in the local area via resources such as the ASHA listserves can provide the clinician with a source of clinical experience to enter into the decision-making equation.

TABLE 7.2   Decision-Making Process Before Using a Treatment Procedure

What are the procedure's stated uses?

To which client/patient population does it apply? Is there documented evidence of its validity for use with a specified population?

To which other populations does it claim to generalize?

Are outcomes clearly stated?

Do publications address this procedure? Is the information published in a peer-reviewed professional journal? Is promotional material the only published source of information?

Does peer-reviewed research support or contradict the stated outcomes or benefits?

What is the professional background of the developers of the procedure?

Are similar procedures currently available? How do they compare in performance and cost?

Have you talked with others who have experience with this procedure? What was their experience? Have you considered posting a query on ASHA's interactive member forum on its website?

Is using this procedure within your profession's scope of practice? Is it within your personal scope of practice (i.e., personal training, competence, experience)?

Have you checked for any ASHA statements or guidelines on this topic?

Based on the factors listed above, is the cost reasonable and justifiable?

What are the potential risks/adverse consequences?

What are the potential benefits?

What is recommended as sufficient training to be considered a qualified user of the technique/procedure? (ASHA, 2004)

In most situations, the speech-language pathologist works within a broader service context that requires coordination and collaboration with practitioners in other disciplines. These interdependencies may vary depending on the specific practice environments, and relate to broader issues such as reimbursement patterns as discussed in Chapters 10, 11, 12, and 13. Thus, it is also critical for the expert clinician to check how other experts perceive speech-language services, and to bring forward evidence that convinces others about the effectiveness of applied treatments. At this point, it is important to have knowledge of practice guidelines developed by groups outside of speech-language pathology. It is also important to understand how practice guidelines for disorders that typically require a multidisciplinary approach, such as autism or stroke, address areas in the domain of the speech-language pathologist.

Practice Guidelines

Practice guidelines were first developed by the Department of Health and Human Services' Agency for Health Care Policy and Research, now the Agency for Health Care Research and Quality (AHRQ; ASHA, 2004a, b, c). AHRQ also funds development of evidence tables for treatments and assessment of the effectiveness, risks, and benefits of technological applications. According to ASHA (2004a, b, c), through concerns about analysis methods, the results of some AHRQ evidentiary analyses have not always been accepted into our field. The expert clinician should follow the publication of practice guidelines and other evidence summaries by groups such as AHRQ and stay abreast of ASHA reactions or responses. Previously accepted practice guidelines from all areas of health care are also available through the National Guidelines Clearinghouse. See Appendix B for information about accessing these resources.

Cochrane Collaboration for Children's Guidelines

The Cochrane Collaboration is another searchable source for published reviews on treatment effectiveness or for guidelines on treatment of a particular disorder. For example, a Cochrane review is available for speech and language treatment for children and adolescents with primary speech and language delay/disorder (Law, Garrett, & Nye, 2004). The review considered the results of 25 randomized controlled trials after a systematic and exhaustive search of the literature. The meta-analysis results suggested that treatment for children with phonological and vocabulary difficulties is effective, but less evidence supported the effectiveness of treatment for children with receptive language difficulties. The effectiveness of intervention for syntactic impairments showed only mixed results. No difference appeared in the effectiveness of treatment administered individually or in groups, but incorporating normal language peers into the intervention had a positive effect, as determined by results across the 25 studies. These broad conclusions based on analysis of 25 well-designed studies can show parents, practitioners of other disciplines, or third-party payers persuasive evidence about the usefulness of certain speech-language pathology services. A report such as the Cochrane review also highlights areas that need additional clinical research. In this case, receptive and syntactical disorders need more research.

TREATMENT FIDELITY AND TREATMENT INTEGRITY

Treatment Fidelity

Treatment fidelity consists of **treatment integrity,** or ensuring that a treatment condition was implemented as planned in a research study (Vermilyea, Barlow, & O'Brien, 1984; Yeaton & Sechrest, 1981), and **treatment differentiation,** ensuring that treatment conditions under study differ sufficiently that we can assume the intended manipulation of the independent variable occurred (Moncher & Prinz, 1991). An important part of treatment fidelity is also replicability. Treatment integrity also measures the reliability of the independent variable in a treatment study. Although researchers in speech-language pathology have been urged to consider, establish, and report treatment integrity in research studies (Hinckley, in preparation; Ingham & Riley, 1998), issues of treatment fidelity and integrity have been rarely acknowledged in speech-language pathology. In contrast, a relatively large scientific literature on treatment integrity has developed in related fields such as education, applied behavior analysis, and psychology.

Any treatment research study involves planning and designing a particular experimental treatment and establishing a protocol. Most include specific training to ensure that individuals administering the treatment under study are consistent and adhere to the experimental protocol. A target treatment may be compared to a control condition (no treatment or a placebo) or an already established treatment. Treatment differentiation helps avoid situations where, if the two treatments are similar in procedure or in the underlying mechanism of change, potential differences between the two treatments may go undetected. When the research study is completed, the reported results should include a sufficient description of the treatment to allow clinicians to apply the treatment, should the evidence support its effectiveness.

In each treatment research study on which we formulate our evidence-based practice, the level of treatment fidelity is critical. Treatments used in clinical research should be described specifically and thoroughly enough to be replicable. Replication allows researchers to accumulate evidence for a particular treatment or treatment protocol, and thus directly contributes to development of practice guidelines.

Treatments described in sufficient detail to be experimentally replicated are also described in sufficient detail to be carried out in clinical practice. Treatment research that fails to specify details of the investigated treatment offers clinicians no guidance in specific procedural decision making. Working from such research, puts clinicians at risk for implementing relatively weak, ineffective, or potentially harmful variations to a treatment protocol.

Another important component of treatment fidelity is treatment integrity, or ensuring that a treatment is actually administered throughout a research study as intended. In a research study, once individuals involved in administering a treatment have been trained, periodic review should follow that confirms that the treatment is being administered reliably. **Therapist drift** is the idea that individuals administering a treatment in a study may unintentionally alter the treatment protocol in small, gradual ways (Peterson, Homer, & Wonderlich, 1982). This gradual shift can change treatment potency, either positively or negatively. In any case, the study outcome ends up associated with the treatment as planned rather than the treatment as actually administered, possibly producing faulty conclusions.

Treatment Integrity

Treatment integrity can be measured in direct or indirect ways (Gresham, 1996). **Direct techniques** include direct observation of planned or randomized research sessions by independent observers, who assess critical components of the treatment protocol for occurrence or nonoccurrence. **Indirect techniques** include self-report by the individual administering the treatment after each session or, in some cases, report by the participant who is receiving the intervention. When researchers apply direct observation of treatment integrity, they can report a percentage of critical components occurring in the sessions sampled as the level of treatment integrity, much as when reporting the reliability of the dependent variable.

How much difference can seemingly small changes in implementation really make to the outcome of a treatment program? A study investigating outcomes of social skills training for students with moderate to severe disabilities provides an example

(McEvoy, Shores, Wehby, Johnson, & Fox, 1990). After the study on outcomes of social skills training was completed, the researchers divided the special education teachers who had participated in the study into two groups: those teachers with the highest treatment integrity and those with the lowest. Students whose teachers were in the high treatment integrity group had superior outcomes to those students taught by teachers with low treatment integrity.

In another education-related example, researchers measured students' performance in a math instructional program with complete and accurate implementation of the intervention and lower levels of integrity (Noell, Gresham, & Gansle, 2002). The math instruction program protocol included systematic prompts to the students to use specified strategies. The study compared the performance of students when they received the prompts 100% of the time as designed, 67% of the time, and 33% of the time, to mimic inconsistent or partial implementation. Students performed significantly better when they received the instructional program with 100% treatment integrity or adherence to the originally designed intervention.

Clinical Decision Making

When we base our clinical decision-making processes on scientific evidence first, then we must be willing to implement a specific treatment program in the same way in which it originally demonstrated its effectiveness. Treatments not administered in the way in which they were used during the accumulation of the evidence might be null and void.

The ASHA Code of Ethics (ASHA, 2003), Principle II, Rule F, states that "Individuals shall ensure that all equipment used in the provision of services . . . is in proper working order and is properly calibrated." Although this rule clearly refers to equipment, its spirit applies to treatment fidelity. Many speech-language pathology interventions forego mechanical devices and rely instead on the clinician's powers of observation and reasoning to make clinical decisions—including treatment decisions—and to carry out an intervention. In that sense, then, the clinician's therapy procedures and skills must be calibrated to the scientific evidence. This means that clinicians using an established treatment should calibrate themselves to the specific procedures that have already demonstrated effectiveness.

ADDITIONAL CONSIDERATIONS: THE NATURE AND AMOUNT OF TREATMENT

Nature of Treatment

An important part of administering an established treatment appropriately is to understand the treatment's action, or how it achieves its potency. Various treatments rely on differing learning mechanisms (for an example pertaining to aphasia therapy, see Hinckley, 2002). In speech-language pathology, some treatments for certain disorders may rely on motor learning theory. Other treatments may rely on different memory subsystems. For example, errorless learning, an established approach with individuals with memory disorder, is lately being applied to aphasia therapy (Fillingham, Hodgson, & Sage, 2003). **Errorless learning** assumes that the procedural memory and learning system is relatively intact in patients who may have an impaired declarative memory system. These patients can learn new procedures or behaviors if allowed to practice the correct response without error. According to errorless learning assumptions, when the learner produces errors, this reinforces the association between the contextual cue and the learner's incorrect response, a negative outcome.

In contrast, spaced retrieval has also been shown effective with patients with cognitive disorders related to stroke or dementia, for learning specific pieces of information, like a room number (Davis, Massman, & Doody, 2001). In **spaced retrieval,** the client is asked about the target information (e.g., "What is your room number?") at varying intervals, beginning frequently and becoming less frequent, as the correct response is given. In this treatment, repetition and reinforcement appear to be the underlying principles of the treatment's action. This treatment could be characterized as error-full learning, because after the clinician requests the target information, the client is likely at the beginning of training to produce one, and maybe many, incorrect responses. The clinician corrects it and asks the client to repeat the correct information. This process is repeated until the client achieves a criterion performance and the interval between trials is increased.

According to the principles underlying errorless learning and spaced retrieval, it does not seem intuitively consistent to mix these two approaches in any way. The two treatments hold competing assumptions about how best to achieve learning and behavior change. Without scientific evidence supporting their combination, the expert clinician's best guess would be to avoid combining them in the treatment program for a single client.

Amount and Duration of Treatment

In addition to understanding the treatment's underlying action, clinicians who apply research to practice must pay attention to other treatment variables such as session length, duration of treatment, frequency of treatment, or other characteristics of the treatment setting. If a body of clinical research shows that a particular treatment is effective, the clinician must know how frequently and for how long to administer the treatment to produce the expected outcome. The relationship of treatment outcome to amount of treatment administered is a **dosage-response curve.** For every treatment there exists a minimum amount of administration below which the treatment produces no effect, and a maximum amount of administration above which more treatment produces no greater effect. Between those two extremes lies the optimal range of treatment amount in which the maximum benefit can be reasonably or typically expected. These are critical factors in an evidence-based, expert practice.

A CLINICAL EXAMPLE

Let us apply the process of EBP to a clinical example. Imagine that a referred client has velopharyngeal impairment due to dysarthria (such as can occur in cerebral palsy or traumatic brain injury).

The clinician must first consider whether or not assessment and treatment of this disorder is within the professional scope of practice. This first step is skipped in most cases because experienced clinicians are likely to know how the kinds of cases typically referred to them fit into the professional scope of practice.

The clinician must also consider whether or not it is within the personal scope of practice. To determine this, the clinician can consult ASHA guidelines, position statements, and knowledge and skills practice policy documents to help determine if his or her previous "education, training, and experience" (from ASHA Code of Ethics, Principle of Ethics II, Rule B) is appropriate for completing a particular clinical protocol.

A search on the ASHA Online Desk Reference reveals established guidelines for oral and oropharyngeal prostheses, which may become an option for such a patient (ASHA, 1993). The guidelines affirm that working with prostheses such as palatal lifts is within the speech-language pathologist's scope of practice and outline the knowledge and skills necessary to complete this kind of clinical work.

Next, the clinician investigates available sources of information for managing velopharyngeal incompetence in dysarthria. Fortunately, ANCDS practice guidelines in this area are available (Yorkston et al., 2001a, b, c).

The ANCDS practice guidelines describe the number of studies available and their basic characteristics, such as number of participants and their etiologies. The practice guidelines provide a decision-making flow chart for velopharyngeal impairment, as well as guidelines for clinical algorithms given particular characteristics of the client. Assessment of velophayrngeal function, including history, physical exam, speech evaluation, and instrumental exam, should produce a diagnosis of velopharyngeal impairment or observation of normal velopharyngeal functioning. Behavioral management techniques focusing on speech production are endorsed over nonspeech practice techniques, based on clinical evidence and expert opinion. The guidelines offer palatal lift fitting procedures and describe behavioral management techniques for those who cannot tolerate or do not succeed with palatal lifts.

Using the World Health Organization (WHO) International Classification of Functioning (ICF) framework (ICF, 2001), the ANCDS guidelines recommend assessment measures that relate to each of the ICF levels. For example, assessing impairment might include acoustic or physiological measurements. Activity limitations could be assessed by intelligibility or listener perceptual ratings. The clinician might assess participation restrictions with self-ratings or measures of quality of life. Thanks to the available practice guidelines, a complete assessment and treatment protocol can be developed for individual clinical practice and management of each case, or more broadly, for the staff in the clinician's practice setting.

THE ROLE OF CLINICAL EXPERTISE

Since the mid-1980s the principles of evidence-based practice have become more prevalent and integrated into all aspects of health care. Producing treatment research and generating practice guidelines take years. It is not surprising, then, that in spite of our best professional efforts we still lack practice guidelines for all disorder categories in speech-language pathology. Nor do we have an evidentiary base that provides guidance under unusual circumstances. Where the foundation of scientific evidence ends for a particular treatment or disorder, the clinician's expertise must take over in making clinical decisions.

There are two broad categories in which the clinician's expertise plays a prominent role in clinical management decisions. First, certain situations may appear subject to available evidence, but individual characteristics or circumstances may challenge the available scientific base. Second, certain clinical problems may have little scientific evidence available.

At the beginning of this chapter, we introduced the clinical situation of an adult with agrammatic aphasia who was also experiencing visual agnosia. Available reviews of the literature synthesize findings across treatment studies for agrammatism (see, for example, Mitchum, 2001). Mitchum suggests that treatment for sentence production in agrammatic aphasia must focus on verb production in sentences, and is typically ineffective if the clinician targets verb retrieval only. The treatment literature also suggests that training of certain complex sentence types will generalize to other, simpler forms (Thompson, Shapiro, Kiran, & Sobecks, 2003). So, the clinician has a good idea of an effective treatment to try for agrammatism.

Two well-documented treatments for agrammatic aphasia have been established with the use of pictured stimuli and the manipulation of printed words. Another literature search generates only one example of a published case of a blind adult with acquired dyslexia and aphasia for Braille (Birchmeier, 1985). As a clinical expert, one must now consider treatment integrity. Significant modification of either one of these two treatments could potentially affect the outcome.

The first choice is to make accommodations that appear not to disrupt the treatment's potential action. If the client knows Braille, or if text stimuli can be presented in raised lettering, then the printed text portions of the established treatments can be adapted to these formats. Adapting pictured stimuli is more challenging, but the clinician might use real objects or small figurines placed in an arrangement that conveys the relationships depicted in the equivalent pictures.

It is important that making such accommodations is not likely to detract from the potency of the original treatment. In the case presented, exact administration of the therapy as recommended was infeasible. Other potential changes to the treatment such as ignoring whole steps because of the client's lack of vision are much more threatening to its effectiveness and could produce a neutral or negative outcome.

Treatment of Rare Conditions

Occasionally clinicians face extremely rare or previously unknown conditions that require complete reliance on clinical expertise. Then, years of previous experience and ongoing monitoring of scientific advances in our profession will yield the biggest payoff. Cases of lightning strike, or management of cognitive-communicative issues in AIDS, or the newly reported cognitive-communicative issues associated with West Nile virus, are examples of rare or newly occurring conditions for which no practice guidelines exist. Practice guidelines in other areas may, particularly for these examples, be directly relevant or appropriate. But at any point a clinician may be at the frontier of an unknown area, with only an unrelated or minimally related scientific past and personal, professional experience as guides. Then, the clinician who has developed expertise via a combination of knowledge, skills, experience, and problem-solving abilities is the one who will rise to the occasion.

Specifically, **professional skills** (Factor 2) such as becoming a critical thinker, gathering information from all sources, and acquiring advanced knowledge in one's primary area of practice will be important when a case lacks sufficient clinical evidence. Clinicians need these skills to implement all aspects of evidence-based practice and to adhere to published treatment criteria and procedures so that they administer only those treatments from which they can reasonably expect benefit.

Problem-solving skills (Factor 3), such as good decision-making ability, good judgment, experience, and ethical conduct also relate to the issues presented in this chapter. In challenging cases as well as seemingly routine ones, clinicians must adhere to basic principles of evidence-based practice and integrate these principles with clinical judgment.

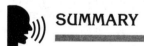 **SUMMARY**

The process of developing clinical expertise relies on continuous development of professional skills and problem-solving abilities. This chapter has described evidence-based practice as one tool with which clinicians continuously monitor their own knowledge base and prepare themselves to make the best decisions about their clients. EBP involves asking appropriate clinical questions and utilizing all possible resources to find relevant information. The clinician must weigh the evidence by relying on disseminated publications or syntheses, or by considering the importance of research design and effect sizes. Additionally, treatment integrity, a general principle of treatment research, equally applies to good clinical practice. We must know that a treatment was implemented consistently in the studies on which we base our clinical decisions, and we must implement the treatment in a similar manner to provide the best possible service and realize the best potential outcome. Where evidence is weak or nonexistent, the expert clinician must rely on individual problem-solving skills, well-developed judgment, and existing knowledge and experience of related situations to make an appropriate judgment consistent with professional ethical conduct.

THOUGHTS FOR EXPLORATION

1. How do professionals apply published research to clinical practice?
2. Why is your clinical experience important to others when you document and publish treatment protocols and outcomes?
3. Why is consistency in daily practice of speech-language pathology important for each client, for each treatment protocol, for each disorder?

REFERENCES

American Speech-Language-Hearing Association. (1993). Position statement and guidelines for oral and oropharyngeal prostheses. *ASHA, 35,* (Suppl. 10), 14–16.

American Speech-Language-Hearing Association. (2003). Code of ethics (revised). *ASHA Supplement, 23,* 13–15.

American Speech-Language-Hearing Association. (2004a). *When evaluating any treatment procedure, product, or program ask yourself the following questions.* Available at: http://www.asha.org/members/evaluate.htm

American Speech-Language-Hearing Association (2004b). *Evidence-based practice in communication disorders: An introduction* (Tech. Rep.). Available at: http://www.asha.org/members/deskref-journals/deskref/default

American Speech-Language-Hearing Association (2004c). *Evidence-based practice: Practice guidelines.* Available at: http://www.asha.org (search for Evidence-based Practice).

Birchmeier, A. K. (1985). Aphasic dyslexia of Braille in a congenitally blind man. *Neuropsychologia, 23,* 177–193.

Cohen, J. (1988). *Statistical power analysis for the behavioral sciences* (2nd ed). Hillsdale, NJ: Erlbaum.

Davis, R. N., Massman, P. J., & Doody, R. S. (2001). Cognitive intervention in Alzheimer disease: A randomized placebo-controlled study. *Alzheimer Disease & Associated Disorders, 15*(1), 1–9.

Drew, R. L., & Thompson, C. K. (1999). Model-based semantic treatment for naming deficits in aphasia. *Journal of Speech, Language, & Hearing, 42,* 972–989.

Fillingham, J. K., Hodgson, C., & Sage, K. (2003). The application of errorless learning to aphasic disorders: Theory and practice. *Neuropsychological Rehabilitation, 13*(3), 337–363.

Frattali, C., Bayles, K., Beeson, P., Kennedy, M., Wambaugh, J., & Yorkston, K. (2003). Development of evidence-based practice guidelines: Committee update. *Journal of Medical Speech-Language Pathology, 11*(3), ix–xviii.

Golper, L. (2001). ANCDS practice guidelines coordinating committee report: Proceedings of the academy of neurologic communication disorders and sciences. *Journal of Medical Speech-Language Pathology, 9,* ix–x.

Gresham, F. (1996). Treatment integrity in single-subject research. In Franklin, R. D., & Allison, D. B. (Eds.), *Design and analysis of single-case research.* Hillsdale, NJ: Erlbaum, 93–117.

Hinckley, J. J. (in preparation). Treatment fidelity, treatment integrity, and treatment differentiation: A tutorial. To be submitted to *Journal of Speech-Language-Hearing Research.*

Hinckley, J. J. (2002). Models of aphasia rehabilitation. In Eslinger, P. (Ed.), *Neuropsychological Interventions.* New York: Guilford Press.

International Classification of Functioning, Disability, and Health. (2001). Geneva: World Health Organization.

Ingham, J., & Riley, G. (1998). Guidelines for documentation of treatment efficacy for young children who stutter. *Journal of Speech-Language-Hearing Research, 41,* 753–770.

Law, J., Garrett, Z., & Nye, C. (2004). Speech and language therapy interventions for children with primary speech and language delay or disorder. *The Cochrane Library,* Issue 4.

McEvoy, M. A., Shores, R. E., Wehby, J. H., Johnson, S. M., & Fox, J. J. (1990). Special education teachers' implementation of procedures to promote social interaction among children in integrated settings. *Education and Training in Mental Retardation, 25,* 267–276.

Mitchum, C. C. (2001). Verbs and sentence production in aphasia: Evidence-based intervention. *Perspectives on Neurophysiology and Neurogenic Speech and Language Disorders, October,* 4–13.

Moncher, F. J., & Prinz, R. J. (1991). Treatment fidelity in outcome studies. *Clinical Psychology Review, 11,* 247–266.

Noell, G. H., Gresham, F. M., & Gansle, K. A. (2002). Does treatment integrity matter? A preliminary investigation of instructional implementation and mathematics performance. *Journal of Behavioral Education, 11,* 51–67.

Peterson, L., Homer, A. L., & Wonderlich, S. A. (1982). The integrity of independent variables in behavior analysis. *Journal of Applied Behavior Analysis, 15,* 477–492.

Robey, R. (April 13, 2004). Levels of evidence. *ASHA Leader,* 5.

Robey, R., & Dalebout, S. (1998). A tutorial on conducting meta-analyses of clinical outcome research. *Journal of Speech, Language, & Hearing Research, 41,* 1227–1241.

Sackett, D. L., Rosenberg, W. M. C., Gray, J. A. M., Haynes, R. B., & Richardson, W. S. (1996). Evidence-based medicine: What it is and what it isn't: It's about integrating individual clinical expertise with the best external evidence. *British Medical Journal, 312,* 711–712.

Sackett, D. L., Straus, S. E., Richardson, W. S., Rosenberg, W., & Haynes, R. B. (2000). *Evidence-based medicine: How to practice and teach EBM.* 2nd ed. Edinburgh: Churchill Livingstone.

Thompson, C. K., Shapiro, L. P., Kiran, S., & Sobecks, J. (2003). The role of syntactic complexity in treatment of sentence deficits in agrammatic aphasia: The complexity account of treatment efficacy (CATE). *Journal of Speech, Language, and Hearing Research, 46,* 591–607.

Vermilyea, B. B., Barlow, D. H., & O'Brien, G. T. (1984). The importance of assessing treatment integrity: An example in the anxiety disorders. *Journal of Behavioral Assessment, 6,* 1–11.

Yeaton, W. H., & Sechrest, L. (1981). Critical dimensions in the choice and maintenance of successful treatment: Strength, integrity, and effectiveness. *Journal of Consulting and Clinical Psychology, 49,* 156–167.

Yorkston, K. M., Spencer, K. A., Beukelman, D. R., Duffy, J., Golper, L. A., Miller, R. M., et al. (2001a). *Practice guidelines for dysarthria: Evidence for the effectiveness of management of velopharyngeal function (Tech. Rep. 1).* Academy of Neurologic Communication Disorders and Sciences.

Yorkston, K. M., Spencer, K. A., Duffy, J. R., Beukelman, D. R., Golper, L. A., Miller, R. M., et al. (2001b). Evidence-based medicine and practice guidelines: Application to the field of speech-language pathology. *Journal of Medical Speech-Language Pathology, 9*(4), 243–256.

Yorkston, K. M., Spencer, K. A., Duffy, J. R., Beukelman, D. R., Golper, L. A., Miller, R. M. et al. (2001c). Evidence-based practice guidelines for dysarthria: Management of velopharyngeal function. *Journal of Medical Speech-Language Pathology, 9*(4), 257–273.

CHAPTER 8

Competence and the Development of Technical Skills

Michael J. Moran

Clinical Competence   The demonstration of appropriate levels of skill, ability, knowledge, and experience required to fulfill the professional role.

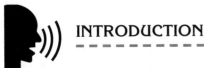 **INTRODUCTION**

Speech-language pathologists across the scope of practice must be prepared to employ technical skills to diagnose and treat speech-language disorders. (See Factor 4 of clinical expertise, technical skills, discussed in Chapter 3.)

How do individuals in need of speech-language services or those who employ speech-language pathologists know that the clinician they select has the competence and technical skills to practice proficiently? Most states require speech-language pathologists to be licensed to practice. However, licensure laws vary widely from state to state. To examine the licensure requirements of every state, we would need 50 separate chapters. We have, fortunately, a universal indicator of competence in speech-language pathology. That indicator is the **Certificate of Clinical Competence (CCC).** The CCC in speech-language pathology indicates that the Council for Clinical Certification (CFCC) has certified the individual in audiology and speech-language pathology. The CFCC is a semi-autonomous organization operating within the American Speech-Language Hearing Association (ASHA). When speech-language pathologists place the letters *CCC* after their names, they tell the world a great deal about their qualifications. They say that they have earned a graduate degree in the field, have demonstrated the knowledge and skills appropriate for entry-level practice in the profession, have passed a national examination in speech-language pathology, have successfully completed a period of supervised on-the-job experience, are bound by ASHA's code of ethics, and have kept abreast of changes in the field through continuing education. Although certification is a valuable indicator of competence, it assures only that the clinician has met a designated threshold for competent practice. Even certified clinicians display varying degrees of expertise in both general abilities and specific disorder areas.

According to the CFCC operating manual (2004), certification has a threefold purpose:

- To promote excellence in speech-language pathology and audiology practice through development and implementation of standards.
- To identify individuals who meet standards necessary to provide clinical services.
- To protect and inform the public by recognizing individuals who meet the certification standards.

TABLE 8.1 The Making of Certification Standards

Year	Activity
1996–1997	ASHA Standards Council (forerunner of the CFCC) developed a plan to identify the experiences required for attaining the critical knowledge and skills necessary for entry-level, independent practice of speech-language pathology.
1997	ASHA commissioned the Educational Testing Service to conduct a skills validation study for the profession of speech-language pathology.
1998	The Standards Council examined information from the following: Skills validation study
	Practice-specific literature (scope of practice statements, position papers, preferred practice patterns, publications of related professional organizations)
	National examination results
	Information obtained from focus group discussions of the future of speech-language pathology (Practice Setting Panel, ASHA Leadership Conference, Multicultural Issues Board, Board of Division Coordinators)
1998	A review of external factors (e.g., demographic factors, changes in health-care and public education service delivery systems and reimbursements, reimbursement regulations, state regulations, legal issues) and consumer groups.
1999	Draft standards constructed.
1999	The draft standards sent out for widespread peer review to groups that include: the ASHA membership, the ASHA leadership, state licensure boards, academic programs, related professional organizations, and consumer groups.
2000	Following the widespread peer review, the final versions of the standards were adopted.
2005	New standards took effect.

HOW CERTIFICATION STANDARDS ARE DEVELOPED

How do certifying organizations such as the CFCC establish the standards they apply to practitioners? To be valid indicators of competence, standards cannot be arbitrarily determined by a small group of individuals sitting around a table. They should reflect input from a broad range of professionals and involve several data-gathering instruments. The background statement that precedes the CFCC standards describes how the most recent certification standards in speech-language pathology were developed, summarized in Table 8.1. Once in place, the standards for the CCC are reviewed periodically to ensure that they continue to reflect the abilities required to practice effectively.

THE PROFESSIONAL COMPETENCIES

The CFCC's most recent certification standards take a form significantly different from earlier versions. Earlier certification standards were mostly "prescriptive," implying that the standards required a minimum number of course credits in certain areas and a minimum number of practicum hours with various disorders. The revised standards, implemented in 2005, are "outcomes based." Rather than simply demonstrating courses completed and accrued practicum hours, applicants for certification must demonstrate knowledge and skills identified in the standards. How students demonstrate the required knowledge and skills is left to the academic programs. The full text of the certification standards appears in Appendix C, and standards for accredited programs are in Appendix D. Table 8.2 lists salient features of the standards for entry-level practice.

Entry-level professionals demonstrate knowledge and skills primarily through academic course work and clinical practicum. The standards indicate that academic course

TABLE 8.2 Salient Features of the Standards for Entry-Level (Novice) Practitioner

✓   A minimum of 75 semester credit hours culminating in a master's, doctoral, or other recognized post-baccalaureate degree initiated and completed in a program accredited by the Council on Academic Accreditation in Audiology and Speech-Language Pathology of the American Speech-Language-Hearing Association.

✓   Demonstrated competencies in knowledge outcomes and skills outcomes.

✓   Practicum experiences that encompass the breadth of the current scope of practice across the age groups, resulting in a minimum of 400 clock hours of supervised practicum (375 direct contact, 25 observation).

✓   Completion of the Speech-Language Pathology Fellowship, which establishes collaboration between the clinical fellow and a mentor and is the equivalent of 36 weeks of full-time practice.

✓   Maintenance of certification requires 30 hours of continuing professional education every three years.

work must be sufficient in depth and breadth to achieve the specified knowledge outcomes and the program of study must address knowledge and skills pertinent to the field of speech-language pathology. A summary of knowledge and skills follows.

KNOWLEDGE OUTCOMES

Basic Science Areas

Applicants for certification must demonstrate knowledge in each of the following areas: biological sciences, physical sciences, mathematics, and social sciences. In a significant change from previous standards, applicants for certification must now demonstrate knowledge in both biological *and* physical sciences. Previous standards required course work in either biological or physical sciences.

Basic Human Communication Disorders and Swallowing Processes

To meet this standard, applicants must demonstrate knowledge of biological, neurological, acoustic, psychological, developmental, and linguistic and cultural bases of basic human communication and swallowing processes. Smoothing the wording of this standard required some sacrifices in clarity. Swallowing disorders have few if any linguistic and cultural bases.

Nature of Speech, Language, Hearing, and Communication Disorders and Differences and Swallowing Disorders

In this area, applicants must demonstrate knowledge about several aspects of the etiology and characteristics of nine specific disorder areas: articulation, fluency, voice and resonance, expressive and receptive language, hearing, swallowing, cognitive aspects of communication, social aspects of communication, and communication modalities. These nine areas have come to be known in the certification jargon as the *big nine*.

Principles and Methods of Prevention, Assessment, and Intervention for People with Communication and Swallowing Disorders

Applicants for certification must demonstrate knowledge regarding prevention, assessment, and intervention in each of the so-called *big nine* areas as cited above. Once again, to make the wording smoother, the standard may cause some confusion. "Communication modalities" is not a disorder. The standard should be interpreted to mean prevention, assessment, and intervention of conditions that may require use of alternative communication modalities.

Additional Knowledge Outcomes

In addition to the knowledge outcomes listed above, applicants for certification must also demonstrate knowledge of the following: standards of ethical conduct, processes used in research and the integration of research principles into evidence-based clinical practice, contemporary professional issues, and knowledge about certification, specialty recognition, licensure and other relevant professional credentials (e.g., state department of education requirements for practice in school settings).

SKILL OUTCOMES

Applicants for certification demonstrate the following skills, categorized as evaluation, intervention, and interaction skills, for each of the *big nine* areas.

Evaluation

Applicants for certification must conduct screening and prevention procedures, collect case history information, select and administer appropriate evaluation procedures, and adapt evaluation procedures to meet client needs. They also interpret, integrate, and synthesize information to develop diagnoses and make appropriate recommendations, complete administrative and reporting functions, and refer patients for appropriate services.

Intervention

Applicants develop and implement setting-appropriate intervention plans with measurable goals, select or develop appropriate materials and instruments for prevention and intervention, measure and evaluate patient performance, and modify intervention plans and materials to meet patient needs. They also complete administrative and reporting functions and refer patients for appropriate services.

Interaction and Personal Qualities

Applicants must demonstrate their ability to communicate effectively with patients, families, and caregivers, recognizing their needs, values, preferred method of communication, and cultural linguistic background. They must collaborate with other professionals in case management, counsel clients regarding communication and swallowing disorders, adhere to the ASHA code of ethics, and behave professionally.

DEMONSTRATION OF KNOWLEDGE AND SKILLS

The knowledge and skills delineated above may appear a bit overwhelming upon first reading. How can an academic program ensure that each student it graduates has not only the knowledge and skills required for certification, but any additional learning the program wishes its students to attain beyond certification standards? To help programs answer this question, the Council on Academic Accreditation has identified six components of good planning programs to ensure that the appropriate knowledge and skills are provided.

Academic and Clinical Curricula Should Include Instruction in the Desired Knowledge and Skills

Although knowledge is generally included in course work, students gain important knowledge in their clinical practicum, too. Specific knowledge areas may be covered in one course or multiple courses, clinical experiences, labs, and so forth. Skills need not be demonstrated only through practicum experience. Other opportunities may include classroom performance or grand rounds demonstrations.

Programs Should Develop Behaviorally Defined Indicators of Knowledge and Skills

These behaviorally defined indicators, also called student learning outcomes, define the acceptable level of success students must exhibit for each type of knowledge and skill. In other words, "What will the student do that indicates achievement or level of mastery?" Like behavioral objectives that students learn to write in clinical practicum, these written student learning outcomes must be observable and measurable. The following are examples of acceptably written student learning behavioral outcomes. Note the use of observable, measurable, action verbs.

- The student will be able to **PERFORM** audiological pure tone screening procedures.
- The student will be able to **IDENTIFY** language disturbances due to dementia.
- The student will be able to **LIST** three benefits of a new augmentative/alternative communication (AAC) device.

The following examples of unacceptable student learning outcomes identify skills and behaviors neither directly observable nor measurable.

- The student will **UNDERSTAND** the importance of cochlear implants.
- The student will become **FAMILIAR** with oral motor therapy techniques.
- The student will **LEARN** about accent reduction.
- The student will **APPRECIATE** the value of a FEES procedure.

Student learning outcomes help educational programs focus on strengths or unique aspects of program offerings. While all accredited programs must include the knowledge and skills identified in the certification standards, the degree to which they cover these requirements depends on each program's goals and objectives.

Programs Should Develop Mechanisms to Assess Student Achievement

Once student learning outcomes have been established; programs must develop one or more mechanisms to assess how well students achieve those learning outcomes. Programs have many ways to assess student learning outcomes, as discussed by Ewell (2001). Whichever they use, effective assessment of student learning outcomes requires good evidence. Ewell indicated that good evidence must incorporate the following.

- *Be comprehensive.* Evidence should cover knowledge and skills taught throughout a program, not just selected portions.
- *Include multiple judgments.* Evidence should come from more than one source. Many graduate programs in speech-language pathology assess knowledge and skills in class and in clinic, in courses and in comprehensive examinations or portfolio evaluations, by faculty and by employers.
- *Include multiple dimensions.* The profession of speech language pathology is ideally suited for multiple judgments. We can judge a person's understanding of concepts of assessment and intervention in classroom and clinic.

TABLE 8.3   Direct vs. Indirect Measures of Student Learning

	Direct Measures	Indirect Measures
Course	Course and homework assignments Examinations and quizzes Standardized tests Term papers and reports Observations of clinical performance Research projects Class discussion participation Case study analysis Rubric (a criterion-based rating scale) scores for writing, oral presentation, and performance Criterion-based rating scale for writing, oral presentations Grades *based on explicit criteria related to clear learning goals*	Course evaluations Percent of class time spent in active learning Number of student hours spent in treatment Number of student hours spent on assignments Grades not based on explicit criteria related to clear learning goals
Program	Capstone projects Pass rates on licensure, certification, or subject-area tests Student publications or conference presentations Employer and internship supervisor ratings of students' performance	Focus group interviews with students, faculty, or employers Course enrollment information Department or program review data Job placement Alumni surveys Student perception surveys Proportion of upper-level courses compared to similar programs at other institutions Graduate school placement rates

Source: From *Student Learning Assessment: Options and Resources.* Middle States Commission on Higher Education. (2003). Reproduced with permission from Middle States Commission on Higher Education.

- *Be a direct measure of student performance.* Evidence should be derived from direct observation or demonstration of student abilities. Although indirect measures of student performance assist some aspects of program evaluation, direct measures tell whether or not a student has mastered a particular learning outcome.

Table 8.3 identifies several direct and indirect methods of measuring student learning outcomes at course and program levels. Note in Table 8.3 that grades generally are inadequate measures of student outcomes. A student may receive a grade of B on a voice disorders test but miss all the questions on causes of vocal nodules; or a student may receive a B in a language disorders class but never adequately demonstrate knowledge of nonstandardized assessment techniques. In both cases the grade masks the student's clear ability in certain knowledge areas and lack of ability in others.

Note that for speech-language pathology certification purposes, applicants may demonstrate knowledge in the basic science areas by course credit, that is, by completing a college/university course in the appropriate area. The question of which courses are acceptable is left to the program in which the applicant received his or her graduate degree. One proviso is that courses used to meet academic requirements for basic human communication and swallowing processes may not be used to meet the basic science requirement. For example, a course in the anatomy of the speech and hearing mechanism cannot be counted in the basic science area *and* in the basic human communication area. As a general rule, courses used to meet the basic science area should be taken outside of programs in communication sciences and disorders.

Assessment of other required knowledge and skills cannot be demonstrated simply by completion of a course. The student must demonstrate the required knowledge and skills.

Programs Must Develop a System to Document Students Progress Toward Achieving Each Knowledge and Skill

Ideally, students should participate in keeping their records of achieving knowledge and skills in addition to the program's record. Programs vary in recordkeeping, but all must answer the following questions:

- What documentation is maintained on each student? What types of experience are credited?
- Who assesses achievements of knowledge and skills?
- When is the decision made?

Questions about the best way to record the attainment of knowledge and skills led the CFCC to develop the Knowledge and Skills Acquisition (KASA) form for program use. Programs are not required to maintain KASAs on each of their students, but they must track student progress.

Programs must do more than simply keep a record of student progress. The data recorded should be shared with students and faculty. Students need to know their progress toward attaining the desired learning outcomes. Faculty need to know how well their students are performing and whether or not their students are attaining the specified learning outcomes. If not, the faculty should determine why not. Ewell (2002) indicated that evidence should be actionable. A student who fails to meet a learning outcome should have some avenue of remediation.

Remediation can be accomplished in various ways. For example, a student clinician who fails to demonstrate the requisite skills with a particular client may be assigned another similar client. A student who fails to master knowledge in a class may have a question that assesses the same area in a comprehensive exam. A student may be assigned extra assignments to demonstrate a particular knowledge or skill as "make-up" or "leveling" work. When many students fail to achieve a learning outcome, that outcome or the steps leading to it should be reevaluated. Programs must answer these questions:

- How will you provide feedback to students, faculty, and clinical supervisors regarding students' level of achievement related to each knowledge and skill?
- How often?

This all relates to another aspect of assessing knowledge and skill required to meet certification standards: the need for both formative and summative assessments. **Formative assessments** are made during the learning process when time remains to remediate or redirect the learner. **Summative assessments** occur at the end of the learning process and indicate whether or not a student has met a particular learning outcome. The following vignette will illustrate formative and summative assessment.

An academic program has a student learning outcome that states, "Students will be able to describe the advantages and disadvantages of the three major types of alaryngeal speech: esophageal, artificial larynx, and tracheo-esophageal puncture." In a graduate-level voice course a student tests poorly on describing the advantages and disadvantages of various types of alaryngeal speech. The professor tells the student, "You have done well enough to pass the course, but you need to review the advantages and disadvantages of alaryngeal speech. I will provide you with some suggested readings." Next semester, the student takes a comprehensive exam required for graduation. The first question on the comprehensive examination is, "Describe the advantages and disadvantages of the three most common types of alaryngeal speech."

In the above situation the test in the graduate-level voice course was a formative assessment. It revealed a weakness addressed by assigning additional readings. The question on the comprehensive examination was a summative assessment. If the student did not know the answer at that point, it was too late for any repair work.

Programs Should Ensure Valid Learning Outcomes

Once student learning outcomes have been identified and a system for assessment of those outcomes is in place, the program must ask, "Are the indicators of achievement and learning goals identified in component 2 appropriate for entry-level practice"? What evidence validated the selected achievement and learning goals? Indicators may include but not be limited to faculty expertise. Other sources of evidence might include best practices documents, scope of practice documents, input from practitioners in the community, and clinical research findings.

Use Learning Outcomes to Continuously Evaluate and Improve the Program

Establishing student learning outcomes and developing methods to assess how well students achieve those outcomes are certainly important aspects of a quality educational program. However, keeping data on student success in attaining those learning outcomes is not enough. Programs must use collected information to identify any problem areas and continuously improve educational procedures. Programs must have a plan and mechanisms in place to evaluate program effectiveness related to student learning outcomes and ability to prepare students to enter professional practice. Evaluation of program effectiveness must be ongoing and systematic. The mechanisms for assessment should include feedback from program alumni, employers of program graduates, and external supervisors. The information collected should help identify patterns of program strengths and weaknesses. There must be a plan to use the information collected to improve the program.

THE CLINICAL FELLOW: BETWEEN STUDENT AND CERTIFIED PROFESSIONAL

Although the knowledge and skills required to graduate from a Council on Academic Accreditation (CAA) accredited program are extensive, they do not, by themselves, prepare an individual to function as an independent professional in speech-language pathology. To demonstrate that level of independence, applicants for the CCC in speech-language pathology must complete a period of supervised professional employment known as the clinical fellowship (CF). According to ASHA's *Certification and Membership Handbook for Speech-Language Pathology* (2000), the clinical fellowship is a transitional phase between graduate-level practicum and independent delivery of services. According to the handbook, inherent in the transition are

- Development of a total commitment to quality speech, language, and hearing services.
- Integration and application of theoretical knowledge gained in academic training.
- Evaluation of individual strengths and limitations
- Refinement of clinical skills.
- Development of clinical skills consistent with the current scope of practice in the profession (p. 31).

Clinical fellowship length varies according to how many hours per week the fellow is employed. If the fellow works 30 or more hours per week (considered full time), the fellowship must last at least 36 weeks. It is possible to fulfill the CF with less than full-time employment; however, the CF period lengthens as follows: employed 25–29 hours per week, CF at least 48 weeks; employed 20–24 hours per week, CF at least 60 weeks; employed 15–19 hours per week, CF must be at least 72 weeks. In most cases, employment of less than 15 hours per week does not qualify for the CF. However, following a 2004 modification of the CF guidelines, students enrolled in doctoral programs and doctoral-level university faculty who have completed the academic course work and clinical practicum requirements for ASHA certification may count weeks with as few as 5 hours of clinical services toward the CF and take up to 48 months to complete the CF.

The person supervising a CF must hold the CCC in speech-language pathology and must have a specified number of contacts with the fellow (at least 18 on-site observations and at least 18 other monitoring activities). The supervisor rates the fellow's performance according to the *Clinical Fellowship Skills Inventory*, an assessment instrument consisting of 18 skill statements related to evaluation, treatment, management, and interaction. The fellow is rated on a five-point scale with 5 representing the most effective performance and 1 representing least effective performance. Twelve of the 18 skills rated on the *Clinical Fellowship Skills Inventory* are considered "core skills." The fellow should receive a rating of at least 3 on each of the core skills to successfully complete the CF.

THE PRAXIS™ EXAM

The Praxis™ series of examinations are developed and validated by Educational Testing Service (ETS), the same organization that produces the Scholastic Aptitude Test (SAT) and the Graduate Record Examination (GRE). The Praxis™ exam in speech-language pathology is one of several subject assessment tests offered as part of the Praxis™ II series. The two-hour examination consists of 150 multiple-choice questions. ASHA collaborates with ETS in construction, validation, and periodic review of the exam. To be eligible for certification, an applicant must achieve a passing score on the Praxis™. The passing score is subject to change as a result of the periodic reviews and validation procedures; however, for the past several years the passing score on the Praxis™ has been 600. Several state licensing agencies and school districts also require the Praxis™ exam, but the passing score for these organizations may differ from that required by the CFCC for certification.

The Praxis™ exam in speech-language pathology was validated for examinees taking the test after the clinical fellowship experience. In spite of this fact, most students choose to take the exam while still enrolled in their graduate program.

Continuing Education

The speech-language pathology profession changes and expands over time. New clinical techniques are developed, research alters our understanding of communication processes and disorders, and our scope of practice expands. Such changes make the field both exciting and challenging. To maintain the competence required for independent practice, speech-language pathologists must continue their education long after they earn their entry-level degree. To maintain certification, practitioners must demonstrate continued professional development. Individuals who hold the CCC in speech-language pathology must accumulate the equivalent of 30 contact hours of professional development every three years. They do this in several ways, described in more detail under Standard VII in Appendix C. Possibilities include attendance at professional meetings and workshops, enrolling in university courses, or self-study videotape, and journal readings. Most states also require continued professional development as part of their license requirements. The number of hours of continuing education and the time period over which those hours must be accrued vary from state to state.

Specialty Recognition

Most speech-language pathologists practice as "generalists." This means that they work with any disorder that falls within the speech-language pathology scope of practice. However the scope has expanded considerably since the early days of the profession. Additionally, our knowledge base regarding the processes and disorders with which we work continues to grow rapidly. As a result many practitioners today agree that it is impossible to be an "expert" in every area of the profession. ASHA, in 1995, initiated a program to recognize speech-language pathologists with advanced knowledge, skills, and experience beyond the Certificate of Clinical Competence: the Specialty Recognition Program. The Council for Clinical Specialty Recognition (CCSR) reviews and approves petitions to establish specialty boards in specific areas of clinical practice. Once approved, a specialty board reviews applications from individual practitioners and confers specialist status on qualified applicants. Individuals who hold specialty recognition identify themselves as a "Board-Recognized Specialist in _____." Participation in a specialty recognition program is voluntary and professionals need not have specialty recognition in an area to practice in it. To date, specialty boards have been established in three areas: child language, fluency disorders, and swallowing and swallowing disorders. Although qualifications for specialty recognition vary among the three specialty boards, each requires extensive experience and professional development beyond certification standards.

Accreditation of Academic Programs

Just as certification shows the public that an individual practitioner has met certain minimum professional qualifications, accreditation is a similar sign regarding academic programs. One requirement for certification is that the applicant graduate from a program accredited by the Council on Academic Accreditation (CAA). The CAA is a semi-autonomous organization within ASHA that sets standards for academic programs. Even people who have been in the field of speech-language pathology for many years sometimes confuse the roles of the CFCC (also a semi-autonomous organization within ASHA) and the CAA, but the two are separate entities. The CAA accredits academic programs, and the CFCC certifies individuals as speech-language pathologists. Accreditation standards serve several purposes:

- Promote excellence in preparing students to enter the profession of speech-language pathology or audiology.
- Protect and inform the public by recognizing programs that meet or exceed accreditation standards.
- Stimulate improvement of programs' educational activities by means of self-study and evaluation. (CAA, 2004, p. 17).

Because this text is designed for students rather than program faculty, we will not go into great detail regarding accreditation standards. We do believe though, that students should understand the bases for judging the quality of an educational program in speech-language pathology. To be accredited by the CAA, an academic program must comply with 31 specific standards organized into five areas. Table 8.4 identifies the standards areas and the kinds of information the CAA looks for in each.

The questions listed in Table 8.4 are answered in two ways. Each program seeking accreditation must submit an application every eight years that addresses the specific standards. After the CAA reviews the application, a team consisting of a practitioner and faculty members from another accredited program make an on-site visit to the program to verify information in the program's application. Each year, programs must file an annual report with the CAA addressing any changes in the program since the last full accreditation review.

TABLE 8.4 Five Areas of Accreditation Standards in Speech-Language Pathology and Factors Evaluated in Each Area

Standard Area	Factors evaluated in the standard area
Administrative structure and governance	Mission, goals, and objectives of the institution, college, and program. The program's student learning outcomes. Does the program conduct on-going and systematic self-evaluation?
Faculty/instructional staff	Is the number and quality of faculty sufficient? Are faculty members adequately prepared for their roles? Do faculty members maintain continued competence?
Curriculum (academic and clinical education)	Does the curriculum include all knowledge and skills required for certification? Is there a mechanism for ensuring that the curriculum is current and is updated as needed? Is the sequence of courses and practicum experiences appropriate? Does the clinical education program include a sufficiently broad range of clients and appropriate supervision? Are ethical, legal, and safety issues covered?
Students	Are students treated fairly, advised regularly, and made aware of all requirements and options?
Program resources	Are the program's financial, physical, and clinical resources adequate to meet the program's goals? Are physical facilities safe and accessible?

WHO RECOGNIZES ACCREDITING ORGANIZATIONS?

Any group or organization can call itself an "accrediting agency." However, for accreditation to be meaningful, the accrediting body should be recognized by an outside group and meet its standards. In the United States, two primary organizations are recognized as accrediting bodies for higher education: The United States Department of Education (USDE) and a private organization, the Council for Higher Education Accreditation (CHEA). ASHA's academic accreditation body (the CAA and its predecessors) began accrediting programs in 1958 and has held USDE recognition continuously since 1967 and from CHEA since 1964. In addition to being a mark of quality, recognition by the department of education enables CAA-accredited programs to establish eligibility to participate in certain federal programs. Accreditation from a recognized accrediting agency is required for participation in federal programs such as the **Individuals with Disabilities Education Act** and the **Rehabilitation Act of 1973,** as amended. CHEA recognition confers academic legitimacy on accrediting organizations, helping to solidify the place of these organizations and their programs in the national higher education community.

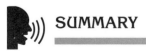 **SUMMARY**

The competencies and skills outlined in this chapter can be viewed as steps on a stairway that speech-language pathologists ascend as they rise from novice to expert. Learning outcomes associated with the basic sciences and normal development courses lay the foundation for obtaining the knowledge of various speech and language disorders. The learning outcomes resulting from disorder courses allow for the emergence of skills further developed in clinical practicum experiences. The skill levels developed in closely supervised university practicum experiences are further elevated in the more independent environment of the clinical fellowship. Certification as a speech-language pathologist, although a worthy accomplishment, is only the first landing on the professional stairway. Certified clinicians continue to elevate their level of knowledge and skill through continuing education in a variety of formats including professional meetings, workshops, university courses, and directed readings. The process of certification ensures that novice speech-language pathologists gain knowledge and skills adequate to practice with at least basic competence. The process of accreditation ensures that academic programs offering entry-level degrees in speech-language pathology provide the appropriate levels of knowledge and skills for initial certification.

THOUGHTS FOR EXPLORATION

1. Explain how the minimal competencies acquired through graduate study and clinical practice provide expected entry proficiency across the profession.
2. How do clinicians build on minimal clinical competencies to establish their individualized specialization and expertise?
3. Which of the areas of competency and skills seems of highest significance to the novice clinician?

REFERENCES

American Speech-Language-Hearing Association. (2000). *Certification and membership handbook: Speech-language pathology.* Rockville, MD: Author.

Council for Clinical Certification in Audiology and Speech-Language Pathology. (2004). *Operating manual.* Rockville, MD: American Speech-Language-Hearing Association.

Council on Academic Accreditation in Speech-Language Pathology and Audiology. (2004). *Operating manual.* Rockville, MD: American Speech-Language-Hearing Association.

Ewell, P. T. (2001). *Accreditation and student learning outcomes: A proposed point of departure.* An occasional paper prepared for the Council for Higher Education Accreditation, Washington, DC.

Ewell, P. T. (2002). CHEA Workshop on Accreditation and Student Learning Outcomes. Chicago, IL. Sept. 25, 2002.

Middle States Commission on Higher Education. (2003). *Student learning assessment: Options and resources.* Philadelphia, PA: Author.

CHAPTER 9

The Influence of Knowledge and Experience on Responding to Diversity in Speech-Language Pathology

Linda I. Rosa-Lugo and Tempii Champion

Diversity   The inclusion of individuals representing a range of demographic characteristics related to ethnicity, religion, national origin, income, education, community, gender or sexual orientation, and associated values, customs, and traditions.

INTRODUCTION

One way to explore **knowledge and experience** of clinical expertise as presented in Chapter 3 is to consider the diversity among American Speech-Language-Hearing Association (ASHA) members in knowledge base, scope of practice, and services to underserved populations. Practitioners need to pursue lifelong learning and experiences with cultures other than their own. In such interactions the clinician needs excellent interpersonal skills to interpret verbal and nonverbal messages from clients and caregivers. Cultural diversity readily recognizes such differences as socioeconomic status, gender preferences, and belief systems. An individual's culture and the clinician's treatment programs incorporate cultural diversity in ethnic groups as well as geographical differences, age, gender, sexual orientation, and educational diversity.

According to Goodenough (1957), **culture** is learned and distinct from one's biological heritage. Culture is the end product of learning. Culture is not a material phenomenon; it does not consist of things, people, behavior, or emotions. Instead, a culture is an organization of people interacting with their environment and each other.

Cultural competence is a multidimensional concept that encompasses cultural awareness, cultural sensitivity, cultural tolerance and an understanding of how the cultural idiosyncrasies of a given population affect their communication interactions, perception of disability, and overall health status (Cross, Bazron, Dennis, & Isaacs, 1989; Isaacs & Benjamin, 1991; Wolf, 2000). Cultural competence reaches well beyond knowing a client's language. Speech, language, and communication are embedded in culture; therefore, one cannot understand a group's communication without understanding the cultural factors that influence its communication (Battle, 2002; Wolf, 1999). Within the human services literature, the most commonly used definition for cultural competence is "the ability of service providers to respond optimally to all children, understanding both the richness and the limitations of the socio-cultural contexts in which children and families, as well as the service providers themselves, may be operating" (Barrera & Kramer, 1997, p. 217).

To attain cultural competence, professionals must acquire pertinent knowledge and apply this knowledge to make appropriate inferences about another's culture (Wolf, 2000; Calderón, Wolf, Baker, & Edelstein, 1998). Most professionals, regardless of their cultural background, require intensive training to maximize their service delivery to diverse populations. Understanding one's own culture is a start, but it does not generalize to all others (Wolf & Calderón, 1999). Cultural competence ultimately includes knowing when to seek cultural advice. By developing these skills, professionals increase their cross-cultural competency.

Research has demonstrated the effects of cultural and social factors on students' learning, especially those from **culturally and linguistically diverse (CLD)** backgrounds (Genesee, 1994; Ogbu, 1992; Ogbu & Simons, 1998; Vygotsky, 1962; Zanger, 1994). We largely define communication within the context of our personal history and the historical, geographic, social, and political issues that bind us to our group. These factors are important in understanding the relationship between individuals and their culture. As Battle (2002) elegantly stated, "Truths are merely perceptions of truth viewed through the prism of culture" (p. xviii).

Attaining cultural competence begins with the individual insights that can foster an awareness of personal value systems. Because speech-language pathologists face a formidable task in providing appropriate services to CLD clients, professionals must examine their attitudes toward diversity and transform any biases that could create difficulties (Coleman & McCabe-Smith, 2000). Professionals must assess their personal values and recognize how these belief systems may influence their clinical practice (Baker, 1995; Banks, 1993; Hidalgo, 1993). Clearly, careful self-analysis should lead to fundamental transformations in beliefs and practices (Cochran-Smith, 1995a, 1995b; Ladson-Billings, 2001; Valli, 1995). Some research-based training programs have encouraged professionals to recognize their biases and to connect them during their professional practices. ASHA has addressed the academic, clinical, and language proficiency competencies of speech-language pathologists through various programs; however, some individuals might consider these issues too challenging to address (Pate, 1992; Peterson & Barnes, 1996; Rosa-Lugo & Fradd, 2000; Sleeter, 1993).

Opportunities for underrepresented individuals to see people of the same racial, ethnic, cultural, or linguistic background participate in valued roles (as teachers, clergy, television cast members, physicians, and child-care workers) is considered important to development of identity and self-esteem (Hains, Lynch, & Winton, 2000). From this perspective, we assume that, in most instances, educational and caregiving settings similar in style, language, and approach to children's home environments are beneficial in assessing and treating CLD individuals (Phillips & Crowell, 1994; National Association for the Education of Young Children, 1996).

Over the years, the profession has stressed the importance of adapting the service delivery process to meet the needs of diverse populations. ASHA is committed to sociocultural diversity throughout the association and professions, particularly in the areas of clinical practice, professional education, and research (ASHA, 1991). This objective recognizes the need to understand cultural diversity in terms of age, gender, sexual orientation, ethnicity, geographical location, and disabilities to provide proper clinical services for certain treatments (Alston & McCowan, 1995; ASHA, 1991; Davis, Brown, Allen, Davis, & Waldron, 1995; Smith, Plawecki, Houser, Carr, & Plawecki, 1991). Service providers must be sensitive to cultural diversity to deliver effective and appropriate treatment (ASHA, 1991).

COMPETENCE

ASHA has recommended academic competencies for speech-language pathologists who work with culturally and linguistically diverse clients to ensure clinician sensitivity to cultural diversity. These competencies include clinical management of CLD populations with communication disorders (ASHA, 1985), linguistic competencies for practicing professionals (ASHA, 1989a, 1998a), guidelines on managing bilingual programs

(ASHA, 1989b), academic competencies for speech-language pathologists working with **English-language learners (ELLs)** who may be diagnosed with communication disorders (ASHA, 1998b), and guidelines on the role of speech-language pathologists in working with clients who speak nonstandard dialects (ASHA, 1983, 2003a).

ASHA's development of checklists to assess one's current level of cultural competence (see ASHA, 2004a) and supplemental reading lists about communication disorders in CLD populations (ASHA, 1995) have been compiled for speech-language. Beginning in 1996, ASHA funded projects on multicultural activities that expand awareness of communication disorders and multiculturalism.

At a recent ASHA legislative council meeting (2004b) several initiatives were proposed to increase (a) awareness of the professions among racial/ethnic minorities; (b) the number of people of racial/ethnic minorities enrolled in academic programs in communication sciences and disorders; (c) the number of racial/ethnic minority members of ASHA; and (d) to ensure that all ASHA members have access to resources to facilitate the acquisition of cultural competency for increasing and improving service delivery to multicultural populations. Many of these initiatives have been advanced for several reasons:

- Demographic changes in the United States (Chavez, 1997; Isaacs & Benjamin, 1991; Lynch & Hanson, 1998; Phillips, 1993).
- Increased interest in cultural understanding in normal and dysfunctional behavior (Battle, 2002; Bebout & Arthur, 1992; Campbell, 1994; Kayser, 1995).
- Ethical and legal requirements for gender, race, and disability equity (Fish, 1986; Gonzalez, Brusca-Vega, & Yawkey, 1997).
- Validation of individuals from underrepresented cultural and linguistic groups (e.g., Barrera & Kramer, 1997; Kappa Delta Pi, 1994; Phillips, 1993).
- Consideration for cultural issues in speech-language acquisition, assessment, and intervention (Kayser, 1995).

CULTURAL DIVERSITY AND SECOND LANGUAGE LEARNING

To ensure that speech-language pathologists are prepared to provide appropriate services, they must be well-informed about culture and its effect on normal behavior and disability (Gopaul-McNicol & Thomas-Presswood, 1998). A major challenge confronting professionals is that normal behavior varies widely among monolingual children. In culturally and linguistically diverse children this variation may appear more complex, especially to the inexperienced professional. What constitutes "normal" and "abnormal" is problematic: certain behaviors are often culturally determined. In working with CLD children, professionals must determine language differences and language disorders in nonnative speakers (Goldstein, 2004; Roseberry-McKibben, 2002). Professionals must be aware that second-language acquisition may cause non-native speakers to experience devaluation of their native culture. Kayser (1995) noted that professionals must be well-informed about second-language acquisition and cultural effects on rehabilitation and education.

Skilled professionals know about cultural diversity and second-language learning and have participated in workshops and conferences in order to diagnose and treat culturally diverse clients. Effective treatment requires expanding our cultural knowledge.

LEGAL AND ETHICAL REQUIREMENTS FOR DIVERSITY

Speech-language pathologists need to recognize ethnic and cultural differences to avoid inappropriate identification and mislabeling of CLD students or biased perceptions against diverse groups. Many organizations such as The Council of Exceptional

Children (CEC), The American Psychological Association (APA), and the American Speech-Language-Hearing Association (ASHA) have developed codes of ethical behavior that address the special needs of CLD students and their families. These organizations have also developed a set of general principles for professionals working with CLD individuals (Gopaul-McNicol & Thomas-Presswood, 1998). For example, recent ASHA code of ethics (2005) revisions address cultural competence of speech-language pathologists. Research (Kritikos, 2003) has indicated that most school-based speech-language pathologists (85%) admitted they lacked competence, even with the help of an interpreter, to assess nonnative speakers' language development (Roseberry-Mckibben and Eicholtz, 1994). However, according to ASHA's code of ethics only certified and fully competent professionals should provide the needed services.

ACQUISITION, ASSESSMENT, AND INTERVENTION

Culture affects every aspect of communication, which makes every clinical encounter a multicultural event (Battle, 2002; Wolf, 1999). Therefore, professionals should consider cultural diversity in every aspect of the discipline. Speech-language pathologists must be encouraged to understand the dimensions of culture and communication and how these influence individuals as well as the clinical environment (Battle, 2002).

COMPETENCE TRAINING

Do speech-language pathologists and audiologists understand the influence of culture on delivery of health-care and educational services? Although the speech-language pathology and audiology professions have demonstrated a commitment to understanding culture's effects on clinical practice and research, as well as the need for education (ASHA, 1991), it is unclear if a majority of speech-language pathologists and audiologists have accepted this challenge. Current efforts to promote cultural diversity may require reevaluation, revision, and greater commitment to achieve cultural competence.

Inadequate cultural preparation in treatment programs produces poor clinical services for CLD populations, making it critical for all professionals to be culturally competent (Association of American Medical Colleges, 1998; ASHA, 2004c; Cohen, 1997). Students, educators, and providers must consider a child holistically (culture, language, family, immigrant status, poverty) and learn effective instructional strategies to meet the needs of diverse clients (Artiles, Harry, Reschly, & Chinn, 2002; McLoyd, 1998; Nieto, 2000; Payne, 2001; Welch, 1998).

Clinicians must use research tools and resources to decide effective strategies for efficient clinical delivery. Speech-language pathologists need to evaluate themselves for cultural biases before they can adjust to the value system of others (Richard & Emener, 2003). Professionals must move beyond simply learning culture-specific information to deliver appropriate treatment (Battle, 2002).

CROSS-CULTURAL COMPETENCE

Lynch and Hanson (1998) describe **cross-cultural competence** as "the ability to think, feel, and act in ways that acknowledge, respect, and build upon ethnic, [socio]cultural, and linguistic diversity" (p. 50). Cross-cultural competence includes attitudes, knowledge, skills, and actions. Currently, many professional organizations require multicultural competencies as part of certification standards. (American Psychological

Association, 1986, 1993; ASHA, 2004c; Council for Exceptional Children, 1996; National Association for the Education of Young Children, 1996; National Council for Accreditation of Teacher Education, 1994).

Human-services literature, designed by Cross et al. (1989), describes a developmental process that spans a six-point continuum and includes "cultural destructiveness, cultural incapacity, cultural blindness, cultural pre-competence, cultural competence, and cultural proficiency" (p. v). Each stage represents a way of responding to diversity. Hains et al. (2000) summarized the work of Cross et al. with the following:

- Cultural destructiveness fosters ethnocentrism and intolerance.
- Cultural incapacity reflects paternalism and condescension.
- Cultural blindness is the denial of diversity.
- Cultural pre-competence is well intentioned but lacks competence.
- Cultural competence is the commitment to implementing cultural diversity and understanding.
- Culturally proficient professionals are trained in this field and are committed to refining their skills through research, seminars, and dissemination.

Cross et al. (1989) suggest individuals can progress toward cultural proficiency through systematic change, training, and personal commitment. Cross-culturally competent individuals support cross-cultural competence/cultural proficiency in every aspect of personal, professional, and organizational functioning (Hains, Lynch, & Winton, 2000).

LANGUAGE DISORDER VERSUS LANGUAGE DIFFERENCE

To differentiate between language disorders and language differences, the speech-language pathologist must know about normal processes of second-language acquisition and how these processes may produce differences that can impede communication. For example, the following are some of the most common processes observed in CLD children learning English as a second language:

- *Interference* is a process in which communicative behavior from the first language (L1) is carried over into the second language (L2; Politzer & Ramirez, 1974).
- *Fossilization* occurs when specific second-language "errors" remain firmly entrenched despite good proficiency in the second language (L2; Naiman, 1974).
- *Interlanguage* refers to a specific second linguistic system resulting from the learner's attempts to produce the target language (Selinker, 1972).
- *Silent period* occurs in learning a second language. Students may go through a silent period of much listening/comprehension and little expressive output (Krashen, 1992).
- *Code-switching* is the alternation between two languages in discourse (Brice & Rosa-Lugo, 2001; Langdon & Cheng, 1992).
- *Language loss* reflects a decrease in use of the first language. It is common for the learner to lose skills in that language as proficiency is acquired in the second language (Anderson, 2004; Schiff-Myers, 1992).

If the clinician does not understand these normal processes, CLD students with communication differences or disorders can be penalized.

ASSESSMENT OF LANGUAGE: ITS DIFFERENCE AND DISORDERS

Because most standardized clinical tests of language abilities often include culturally biased items, the clinician must carefully assess children from culturally diverse backgrounds to determine which children require language intervention for optimal levels of language development and which children have normal development but fall below the published mean on one or more standardized tests. This problem is compounded when children use a nonstandard dialect at odds with the test.

Professionals must recognize diverse cultural performance to make accurate diagnoses and deliver effective instruction and intervention. Given the ongoing overrepresentation of children from culturally diverse backgrounds in speech-language pathology caseloads and in special education classes, one could argue that current practices have failed to accurately distinguish clinical from nonclinical populations (Harry, 1992; Seymour, Bland-Stewart, & Green, 1998).

We cannot ignore widespread failure in evaluating children who require treatment. Although the special-needs child differs from the normal child, there are, nevertheless, important similarities with respect to the context in which their learning occurs as well as the curricular demands they both must face. Indeed, the curricular demands determine the academic preparation and skills required of both normal and special needs children. For this reason, factors that affect "normal" children also influence children with special needs, but to an even greater degree. One must gain an understanding of these factors to adapt and create appropriate instructional strategies. Thus, assessment and treatment strategies must relate to expectations of learning within the academic program.

Clinicians often use more than one type of assessment to ascertain if a child has a language difference or a language disorder. These assessments may include standardized measures, dynamic assessment measures, language sampling, and criterion referenced assessment instruments. Often, standardized tests are biased toward Standard American English (SAE) speakers, which makes them problematic for use with children who speak African American English (AAE).Using a variety of tests may help overcome the weaknesses or biases in any one test.

Wilson and Wilson (cited in Musselwhite, 1983) propose that the following five questions should guide clinicians in their assessment and use of standardized measures with African American children:

1. What is the relationship between the norm sample and the client?

2. What is the relationship between the child's experience and test content areas?

3. What is the relationship between the dialect being tested and the child's dialect dominance?

4. Will the test language penalize a non-standard-speaking child by use of idiomatic or metaphoric language?

5. Is the child penalized for a particular pattern of learning or style of problem solving?

The use of these questions as guidelines in assessing culturally and linguistically diverse children does not guarantee the test used will be free of bias. Many researchers (Champion, 2003; Taylor & Payne, 1983; Washington & Craig, 1992; Washington & Craig, 1999) have studied different assessment instruments and their uses with minority children and found that, as a result, many minority children scored lower than the mean. These findings suggest that standardized tests should not be the sole criterion for determining eligibility for speech and language therapy.

Dynamic assessment, used as a measure of prognosis in children from disordered populations (Goldman & Fristoe, 1986), probes the capability for approximating or using correct linguistic forms using various methods of support. For example, the child receives nonverbal and imitative prompts to determine whether un-acquired forms can be elicited. If forms are produced under elicitation, this suggests that the children possess knowledge of the target and that knowledge could be used to establish spontaneous use of the language forms. Conversely, if a child is not stimulable, this indicates a poorer prognosis as the child evidently has insufficient knowledge of the language form under study to produce the structure even with extensive support from the clinician.

Another way to assess children is to obtain a representative language sample. Clinicians can use narrative or language samples to gather more information of the child's language ability. The clinician should analyze the features (i.e., grammar, syntax, phonology) that AAE speakers and SAE speakers share. Clinicians should know and use appropriate methods of analysis (i.e., t-units, c-units) to assist in formulating appropriate statements and recommendations of a child's language abilities.

Criterion-referenced testing compares a child's performance with criteria for acceptable responses (Terrell & Jackson, 2002). One criterion-referenced measure is Stockman's (1996) Minimal Competency Core. This measure assesses a child's language abilities with criteria set by other children of the same age and dialect use. Seymour, Roeper & deVilliers (2003) have also developed a criterion-referenced screening and assessment test known as the Diagnostic Evaluation of Language Variation (DELV). This measure distinguishes linguistic differences and language disorders. These instruments are examples of measures designed to reduce the over-identification of minority children for speech and language services.

INTERVENTION FOR CHILDREN

Barriers to providing quality educational services to diverse children discussed in the literature include ethnocentric attitudes of professionals; low expectations and negative attitudes toward minority students, their families, and communities; lack of professional training regarding cultural and linguistic diversity; use of biased test measures that result in misdiagnosis; educational materials and curricula that do not incorporate multiculturalism; and inappropriate and inadequate instructional techniques (Campbell, 1996; Ford, 1992; Gay, 1993; Ogbu, 1982). The speech-language pathologist plays a key role in educational outcomes. He or she must construct intervention goals and use intervention techniques that reflect the child's needs and the family's cultural values. Campbell, addressing service delivery options and approaches, notes that with appropriate knowledge and training, speech-language pathologists can work collaboratively with educators to meet the needs of minority children with communication disorders.

According to data from the 2000 U.S. census, approximately 47 million individuals living in the United States speak a language other than or in addition to English (U.S. Bureau of the Census, 2000). Of this 47 million, almost half (45%) report that they speak English "less than very well." Almost 60% of this group (28.2 million) report Spanish as the language they use other than or in addition to English.

The growing population of ELLs in U.S. schools has been well documented. According to the most recent demographic analyses, students who speak a native language other than English represented 9.6% of the school-age population in 2001 (Kindler, 2002). The number of ELL students has increased by more than 95% in the past 10 years, while the school-age population itself has grown by less than 12% (Padolsky, 2002). Although more than 400 languages have been identified in the school-age population, Spanish is the most frequently spoken language, representing 79% of the ELL population (Kindler, 2002).

The extent to which non-native speakers master the English language has educational and economic implications. It also has implications for professionals who work with school-age children and strive to provide appropriate clinical services. To ensure appropriate services for this group requires familiarity with selected studies that explain the history of the first language in the Americas, its general and dialect-specific features, and acquisition of English as a second language (Chang-Rodríguez, 1991; Frago Gracia, 1996; Barrutia & Terrell, 1982; Bedore, 1999; Hakuta, 1994; Krashen, 1981; Molesky, 1988; Goldstein, 2004).

A SHARED KNOWLEDGE BASE

Professionals must share a common philosophy and knowledge base relative to education of students learning English. The rapid growth of CLD students diagnosed with speech and language impairments has greatly challenged the profession of communication disorders. Current research has provided the profession with information on related issues to better understand CLD students with special needs. A primary challenge faced by speech-language pathologists who work with school-age CLD students is appropriate, accurate identification of these students.

Many children struggle with learning English for a variety of reasons. Professionals often treat the fact that a child speaks a language other than English as a problem, despite studies that suggest that a student's native language can be an asset (Collier, 1995; Cummins, 1994; 1996; Gandara, 1995; Soto, 1993; Zentella, 1997). The most common belief for children not learning English quickly and proficiently is that the child has a language disorder. When these children fail to perform well in the classroom, speech-language pathologists often must determine whether there is a language disorder or a language difference.

ASSESSMENT

Students learning English suffer where appropriate assessment instruments and professionals trained to conduct culturally and linguistically relevant educational assessments are scarce (Ortiz, 2001, 2002; Valdés & Figueroa, 1996). The speech-language pathologist must be competent in assessing proficiency in the native language and English. The problematic variables of native-language loss and normal language development in learning a second language make determining the presence of a speech or language disorder difficult (Kayser, 2002). Assessing competence in the linguistic characteristics of a language requires a speech-language pathologist knowledgeable about the language's linguistic features and normal development of these features in the language.

INTERVENTION

Clinicians often ask when diagnosing a bilingual child with a communication disorder, "In which language should the intervention be provided?" With the paucity of research studies and the lack of a theoretical framework in our discipline, well-intentioned clinicians often have forged ahead and made decisions on language choice based on anecdotal evidence, bias, or subtle school policies that suggest that to be successful in school and society it is best to expose a child to one language only.

Although it is often recognized that systematic exposure to two languages may not cause a language disorder, it is more commonly believed that use of two languages can exacerbate an already existing problem. Discussions on language dominance, language proficiency, parental preferences, preservation of a home language, bilingual language stability over time, language importance, and the negative consequence of discontinuous language use reinforce the notion that a single language is always best for the child with a language disorder.

In light of current research in all domains of language development and disorders, Goldstein (2004) suggests that the new question should be how can clinicians structure the language of intervention to ensure gains in both languages for bilingual children with language disorders. Currently, no direct evidence indicates that language-impaired children who receive continuous input in two languages fare worse than monolingual children with a similar impairment. As a result, the clinician may remain reluctant to support development in both languages and implement appropriate, individualized clinical intervention programs.

EDUCATION AND LEARNING: IMPLICATIONS FOR SPEECH-LANGUAGE PATHOLOGISTS

Learning Styles in Culturally and Linguistically Diverse Students

Evaluating learning styles to explain why CLD students often experience academic and linguistic challenges has been subject to debate for decades. In 1983, the National Task Force on Learning Style and Brain Behavior offered the following definition of learning style:

> Learning style is that consistent pattern of behavior and performance by which an individual approaches educational experiences. It is the composite of characteristic cognitive, affective, and physiological behaviors that serve as relatively stable indicators of how a learner perceives, interacts with, and responds to the learning environment. It is formed in the deep structure of neural organization and personality [that] molds and is molded by human development and the cultural experiences of home, school and society. (Keefe & Languis, 1983, p. 1)

This definition emphasizes "cultural experiences of home, school, and society" and has become the basis for research into the nature of learning styles in CLD children (Swisher, 1993). While evidence may point to a relationship between cultural and learning styles, there is also great concern that characterizing learners from particular CLD backgrounds as having specific learning styles may result in discriminatory practice or excuses for academic failure (Swisher, 1993). For example, studies (Ramirez & Castaneda, 1974; Witkin, 1967) have noted cultural, verbal, and nonverbal communication differences that can influence the case history interview, counseling, testing and intervention process with individuals from CLD backgrounds (Swisher, 1993). A clinician who misunderstands and misinterprets the individual's communication differences can seriously jeopardize rapport with the client. Likewise, clinicians unfamiliar with these differences may inadvertently mistake certain communication behaviors as signs of disorder. Differences in learning style preference can also affect the testing process and lead to misdiagnosis as well as inappropriate treatments. Therefore, clinicians to recognize communicative behaviors, learning styles (e.g., field-dependent vs. field-independent) and approaches CLD students take to learning. These may reflect a preference for shared-group learning or decision making rather than for independent learning (Ramirez & Castaneda, 1974; Witkin, 1967).

EDUCATION

A particularly disturbing finding by the National Research Council (2002) is that children of minority status are over-represented in certain categories of special education. This is especially apparent for African American males in high-incidence categories such as mental retardation and emotional disturbance. The commission found several factors responsible for this over-representation, including reliance on IQ tests that reflect known cultural biases, behavioral characteristics associated with the cultural context in which a child is raised, and professionals unprepared to work with CLD individuals (U.S. Department of Education, 2002).

Several researchers have investigated this disproportionate representation of CLD students in special education and have developed theories such as the Deficit-Deprivation Theory and the Theory of Cultural Discontinuity to explain this phenomenon (Gould, 1981; Ladson-Billings, 2001; Rosenthal & Jacobson, 1968; Spindler, 1987). Specific cultural perspectives that may affect minority children include the following:

- Minority children have distinctly different cultures with unique dialects and child-rearing practices (Field & Widmayer, 1981; Quinn, 1995).
- America's schools do not recognize or utilize minority students' competencies for teaching, learning, and testing (Genesee, Paradis, & Crago, 2004; Goldenberg, 2003).
- Overrepresentation of minority children in special education relates directly to cultural discontinuity between students and teachers, home and school environment, curriculum and learning (Artiles et al., 2002; Nieto, 2000).
- Assessment instruments and practices used to evaluate minority students are inherently biased (Kamhi, Pollock, & Harris, 1996; Roseberry-McKibben, 2003).

HOME-SCHOOL/CLINIC MISMATCH

When educators understand that culture provides a context for teaching and learning for all students, they will recognize that differences between home and school cultures can pose challenges for both educators and students (García & Guerra, 2004). Moreover, students' success and failure are considered results of a match (or mismatch) between the learning environment and their learning needs and characteristics (García, Wilkinson, & Ortiz, 1995).

The theory of cultural discontinuity suggests a mismatch between the home culture of students of color and the school culture. Children are socialized into language through everyday activities and experiences with peers and adults. They learn how to think about, talk about, and use language before entering school (Heath, 1983). This classroom use of language may conflict with the language used in the home and/or clinical setting (Ladson-Billings, 2001). Therefore, it is important for the clinician to be aware of the characteristics of the language(s) their clients use and assess these appropriately.

It is important to value the language experiences of CLD individuals. For example, in selecting materials and strategies to work with CLD clients, clinicians should question if these materials and/or strategies are based on middle-class values and norms. A study by McCarthy (1997) found that teachers had more information about middle-class students than about lower-class students from CLD backgrounds, resulting in a curriculum more closely tied to the home practices of middle-class families. To emphasize this point, in 1990, Rosa-Lugo worked in a home health-care setting. During a therapy session with a young child of the Hasidic religion focusing on the correct production of /kl/, she presented a picture of Santa Claus to elicit a targeted response. To her dismay, this picture failed to elicit the target response, and in fact the child failed to recognize the character. That incident taught Rosa-Lugo two important lessons: do not assume that everyone celebrates Christmas and select materials that reflect the individual's culture reality.

TEACHER EXPECTATIONS

Research has suggested that teacher expectations contribute to underachievement of CLD learners and contribute significantly to the quality of their learning opportunities (Gay, 2000). Like so many other aspects of teaching, the expectations of professionals working with CLD children can become a self-fulfilling prophecy. Winfield (1986) describes four categories of teachers in urban schools: tutors, general contractors, custodians, and/or referral agents. **Tutors** are teachers who expect children to achieve and who take responsibility for their students' achievement; **general contractors** believe children can achieve with the help of teacher resources outside the classroom; **custodians** do not believe children can achieve and so direct their efforts toward maintaining a child's current achievement level; and **referral agents** try to refer as many children as possible to special education (Champion, 2003). The expectations of professionals who work with CLD children can contribute to positive learning experiences or their attitudes can lead to negative beliefs resulting in low expectations and underachievement. It is imperative that speech-language pathologists who work with CLD children think about their attitudes and expectations—their beliefs and attitudes affect student performance through curriculum selection and instructional practices.

CULTURALLY RELEVANT PEDAGOGY

Ladson-Billings (2001) has described **culturally relevant pedagogy** as one that empowers students intellectually, socially, emotionally, and politically through the use of cultural referents to impact knowledge, skills, and attitudes. These cultural referents are essential aspects of the curriculum and not merely devices for bridging or explaining the dominant culture. Culturally responsive pedagogy facilitates achievement for all students. In a culturally responsive classroom, effective teaching and learning occurs in a culturally supported, learner-centered context, whereby the strengths students bring to school are recognized, encouraged, and utilized to promote student achievement. Culturally responsive pedagogy comprises three dimensions: institutional, personal, and instructional. The *institutional dimension* reflects the administration and its policies and values. The *personal dimension* refers to the cognitive and emotional processes teachers must engage in to become culturally responsive. The *instructional dimension* includes materials, strategies, and activities that form the basis of instruction (Champion, 2003). All three dimensions interact significantly in the teaching and learning process and are critical to understanding the effectiveness of culturally responsive pedagogy (Richards, Brown, & Forde, 2004). Using a culturally relevant pedagogy may close the gap between home and school cultures and maintain a client's cultural integrity while achieving success.

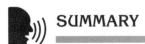 **SUMMARY**

We began this chapter discussing the importance of the individual as a key factor in providing effective therapy. We highlighted the importance of cultural competence and the responsibility of cultural self-assessment. Amassing knowledge and experience with clients from different cultures are essential in becoming a culturally competent speech-language pathologist. Speech-language pathologists must avail themselves of training and education (e.g., staff development, conferences, workshops, courses) to acquire skills and knowledge if they are to meet the service delivery needs of our expanding and diverse population.

Speech-language pathologists working with culturally and linguistically diverse students also need to reflect on how cultural differences may affect student learning and language use. The languages and dialects students bring with them should form an explicit part of the teaching and learning process if we are to convey the message that cultural and linguistic diversity is highly regarded in our multicultural society. Rather than viewing cultural and linguistic diversity as a deficit, professionals need to see it as an asset on which to build additional learning. These concepts transcend all practice settings. Knowledge of the principles of cultural and linguistic diversity is a sign of significant professional expertise. Speech-language pathologists must continue to reflect on and explore their beliefs, skills, and competencies. Those who commit themselves to such professional empowerment will become more effective in culturally relevant clinical practices in communication disorders.

THOUGHTS FOR EXPLORATION

1. What is your level of competence for working with clients and caregivers from other cultural backgrounds?
2. Debate the "culture is innate versus learned" question.
3. What are the dangers of over-generalizing your knowledge of cultural differences?
4. Think about ways in which confrontations between cultures have influenced history. How might similar encounters influence clinical interactions between clinicians and clients/caregivers from different cultures?

REFERENCES

Alston, R. J., & McCowan, C. J. (1995). Perception of family competence and adaptation to illness among African-Americans with disabilities. *Journal of Rehabilitation*, 27–32.

American Psychological Association (1986). *Accreditation handbook* (rev. ed.). Washington, DC: APA Committee on Accreditation and Accreditation Office.

American Psychological Association. (1993). Guidelines for providers of psychological services to ethnic, linguistic, and culturally diverse populations. *American Psychologist*, *48*, 45–48.

American Speech-Language-Hearing Association. (1983, September). Social dialects. *ASHA, 25*, 23–27.

American Speech-Language-Hearing Association (1985). Clinical management of communicatively handicapped minority language populations. *ASHA, 27*(6), 29–32.

American Speech-Language-Hearing Association. (1989a). Bilingual speech-language pathologists and audiologists. *ASHA, 30*(5), 93.

American Speech-Language-Hearing Association. (1989b). Managing a bilingual program. *ASHA, 30*(1), 40–41.

American Speech-Language-Hearing Association. (1991). Multicultural Action Agenda 2000. *ASHA, 33*(5), 39–41.

American Speech-Language-Hearing Association. (1995). *Reading lists on multicultural populations for independent study.* Rockville, MD: Author.

American Speech-Language-Hearing Association Joint Subcommittee of the Executive Board on English Language Proficiency. (1998a). Students and professionals who speak English with accents and nonstandard dialects: Issues and recommendations. Position statement and technical report. *ASHA, 40* (Suppl. 18).

American Speech-Language-Hearing Association. (1998b). Provision of English-as-a-second-language instruction by speech-language pathologists in school settings. (Position statement and technical report). *ASHA, 40* (Suppl. 18).

American Speech-Language-Hearing Association. (2003). Technical report: American English dialects. *ASHA Supplement* 23.

American Speech-Language-Hearing Association. (2004a). *Self-assessment for cultural competence.* Retrieved October 24, 2004, from http://www.asha.org/about/leadership-projects/multicultural/self.htm#ccc

American Speech-Language-Hearing Association. (2004b). *ASHA legislative council meeting CLD focused initiative update.* Retrieved October 24, 2004, from http://www.asha.org/NR/rdonlyres/81F58D5C-33BD-443D-8FF2-927E36DF6BDD/0/VickiCLDFocusedInitiative.pdf

American Speech-Language-Hearing Association. (2004c). *Speech-language pathology competencies.* Retrieved October 24, 2004, from http://www.asha.org/members/slp/competencies/

American Speech-Language-Hearing Association. (In press, 2005). Cultural competence. *ASHA Supplement* 25.

Anderson, R. (2004). First language loss in Spanish-speaking children. In B. Goldstein (Ed.) *Bilingual language development & disorders in Spanish-English speakers* (pp. 187–211). Baltimore, MD: Paul H. Brookes.

Artiles, A. J., Harry, B., Reschly, D. J., & Chinn, P. C. (2002). Over-identification of students of color in special education: A critical overview. *Multicultural Perspectives*, *4*(10), 3–10.

Association of American Medical Colleges. (February, 1998). Teaching and learning of cultural competence in medical school. *Contemporary Issues in Medical Education*, *1*(5) 1–2.

Baker, C. (1995). *Attitudes and language.* Clevedon, Avon, UK: Multilingual Matters.

Banks, J. A. (1993). Education and cultural diversity in the United States. In A. Fyfe & P. Figueroa (Eds.), *Education for cultural diversity: The challenge for a new era* (pp. 49–68). New York: Routledge.

Barrera, I., & Kramer, L. (1997). From monologues to skilled dialogues: Teaching the process of crafting culturally competent early childhood environments. In P. J. Winton, J. McCollum, & C. Catlett (Eds.), *Reforming personnel preparation in early intervention: Issues, models, and practical strategies* (pp. 217–251). Baltimore, MD: Paul H. Brookes.

Barrutia, R., & Terrell, T. (1982). *Fonética y fonología Españolas [Spanish phonetics and phonology].* New York: Wiley.

Battle, D. (Ed.) (2002). Communication disorders in multicultural populations (3rd ed.). Newton, MA: Butterworth-Heinemann.

Bebout, L., & Arthur, B. (1992). Cross-cultural attitudes toward speech disorders. *Journal of Speech and Hearing Research, 35*(1), 45–52.

Bedore, L. (1999). The acquisition of Spanish. In O. Taylor & L. Leonard (Eds.), *Language acquisition across North America,* (pp. 157–208). San Diego: Singular.

Brice, A. & Rosa-Lugo, L. (2001). Codeswitching and codemixing in two classrooms: A bridge or barrier between two languages [Monograph]. *Multiple Voices for Ethnically Diverse Exceptional Learners.* 4(1), 1–12.

Calderón, J. L., Wolf, K. E., Baker, R. S., & Edelstein, R. A. (1998). A model for ethnomedical science education. A seminar presented at the Association for the Behavioral Sciences and Medical Education 28th Annual Meeting, Jackson Hole, WY.

Campbell, L. R. (1994). Learning about culturally diverse populations. *ASHA, 36*(6), 40–41.

Campbell, L. R. (1996). Issues in service delivery to African American children. In A. Kamhi, K. Pollock, & J. Harris (Eds), *Communication development and disorders in African American children,* (pp. 73–93). Baltimore, MD: Paul H. Brookes.

Champion, T. (2003). *Understanding storytelling among African American children: A journey from Africa to America.* Mahwah, NJ: Erlbaum.

Chang-Rodríguez, E. (1991). *Latinoamérica, su civilización y su cultura [Latin America, her civilization and culture].* New York: HarperCollins.

Chavez, J. A. (1997). Preparing special education teachers and leaders for our diverse schools. *Division for Culturally and Linguistically Diverse Exceptional Learners (DDEL) News, 7*(2), 6.

Cochran-Smith, M. (1995a). Color blindness and basket making are not the answers: Confronting the dilemmas of race, culture, and language diversity in teacher education. *American Educational Research Journal, 32,* 493–522.

Cochran-Smith, M. (1995b). Uncertain allies: understanding the boundaries of race and teaching. *Harvard Educational Review, 65,* 541–570.

Cohen, J. (1997). Finishing the bridge to diversity. *Journal of Academic Medicine, 72,* 103–107.

Coleman, T. J., & McCabe-Smith, L. (2000). Key terms and concepts. In T. J. Coleman, *Clinical management of communication disorders in culturally diverse children* (pp. 3–12). Needham Heights, MA: Allyn & Bacon.

Collier, V. (1995). *Promoting academic success for ESL students: Understanding second language acquisition at school.* Elizabeth, NJ: New Jersey Teachers of English to Speakers of Other Languages—Bilingual Educators.

Council for Exceptional Children. (1996). *What every special educator must know: The international standards for the preparation and certification of special education teachers* (2nd ed.). Reston, VA: Author.

Cross T., Bazron, B., Dennis, K., & Isaacs, M. (1989). *Towards a culturally competent system of care,* Vol. 1. Washington, DC.: Georgetown University Child Development Center, CASSP Technical Assistance Center.

Cummins, J. (1994). Knowledge, power, and identifying teaching English as a second language. In F. Genesee (Ed.), *Educating second language children: The whole child, the whole curriculum, the whole community* (pp. 103–125). New York: Cambridge University Press.

Cummins, J. (1996). *Negotiating identities: Education for empowerment in a diverse society.* Ontario, CA: California Association for Bilingual Education, 73.

Davis, I. J., Brown, C. P., Allen, F., Davis, T., & Waldron, D. (1995). African-American myths and health care: The sociocultural theory. *Journal of the National Medical Association, 87*(11), 791–793.

Field, T. M., & Widmayer, S. M. (1981). Mother-infant interactions among lower SES Black, Cuban, Puerto Rican, and South American immigrants. In T. M. Field, A. M. Sostek, P. Vietze, & P. H. Leiderman (Eds.), *Culture and early interactions* (pp. 209–242). Norwood, NJ: Erlbaum.

Fish, D. (1986). Legal issues affecting the delivery of services to minorities. In F. Bess, B. S. Clark, & H. R. Mitchell, (Eds.), *Concerns for minority groups in communication disorders* (pp. 85–88). Rockville, MD: American Speech-Language-Hearing Association.

Ford, B. A. (1992). Multicultural education training for special educators working with African American youth. *Exceptional Children, 59*(2), 107–114.

Frago Gracia, J. (1996). Formación del Español de América [Formation of American Spanish]. In M. Alvar (Ed.), *Manual de dialectología Hispánica: El Español de America* (pp. 11–23). Barcelona, Spain: Ariel.

Gandara, P. (1995). *Over the ivy walls: The educational mobility of low-income Chicanos.* Albany: SUNY Press.

García, S. B., & Guerra, P. L. (2004). Deconstructing deficit thinking: Working with educators to create more equitable learning environments. *Education and Urban Society, 36*(2), 150–168.

García, S. B., Wilkinson, C. Y., & Ortiz, A. A. (1995). Enhancing achievement for language minority students: Classroom, school, and family contexts. *Education and Urban Society, 27,* 441–462.

Gay, G. (1993). Ethnic minorities and educational equality. In J. A. Banks & C. A. McGee Banks (Eds.), *Multicultural education: Issues and perspectives* (2nd ed., pp. 171–194). Boston: Allyn & Bacon.

Gay, G. (2000). *Culturally responsive teaching: Theory, research, and practice.* New York: Teachers College Press.

Genesee, F. (Ed). (1994). *Educating second language children: The whole child, the whole curriculum, the whole community.* New York: Cambridge University Press.

Genesee, F., Paradis, J., & Crago, M. (Eds.). (2004). *Dual language development and disorders.* Baltimore, MD: Paul H. Brookes.

Goldenberg, C. (2003). Making schools work for low-income families in the 21st century. In S. B. Neuman & D. K. Dickinson (Eds.), *Handbook of early literacy research* (pp. 211–231). New York: Guilford Press.

Goldman, R., & Fristoe, M. (1986). *Goldman-Fristoe Test of Articulation.* Circle Pines, MN: American Guidance Service.

Goldstein, B. (2004). *Bilingual language development & disorders in Spanish-English speakers.* MD: Paul H. Brookes.

Gonzalez, V., Brusca-Vega, R., & Yawkey, T. (1997). Assessment and instruction of culturally and linguistically diverse students who are at-risk of learning problems. Needham Heights, MA: Allyn & Bacon.

Goodenough, W. (1957). *Cultural anthropology and linguistics.* University Monograph Series on Language and Linguistics, No. 9, 167.

GoPaul-McNicol, S., & Thomas-Presswood, T. (1998). *Working with linguistically and culturally different children.* Needham Heights, MA: Allyn & Bacon.

Gould, S. J. (1981). *The mismeasure of man.* New York: Norton.

Hains, A., Lynch, E., & Winton, P. (2000, October). *Moving towards cross-cultural competence in lifelong personnel development. A review of the literature.* (Tech. Rep. 3). CLAS: The Early Childhood Research Institute on Culturally and Linguistically Appropriate Services. Retrieved October 24, 2004, from http://www.clas.uiuc.edu/techreport/tech3.html

Hakuta, K. (1994). Distinguishing among proficiency, choice, and attitudes in questions about language for bilinguals. In G. Lamberty & C. Garcia Coll (Eds.), *Puerto Rican women and children: Issues in health, growth and development* (pp. 191–209). New York: Plenum Press.

Harry, B. (1992). *Cultural diversity, families, and the special education system.* New York: Teachers College Press.

Heath, S. B. (1983). *Ways with words: Language, life and work in communities and classrooms.* New York: Cambridge University Press.

Hidalgo, N. M. (1993). Multicultural teacher introspection. In T. Perry & J. W. Fraser (Eds.), *Freedom's plow: Teaching in the multicultural classroom* (pp. 99–106). New York: Routledge.

Isaacs, M., & Benjamin, M. (1991). Towards a culturally competent system of care (Vol. 2). *Programs which utilize culturally competent principles.* Washington, DC: Georgetown University Child Development Center, CASSP Technical Assistance Center.

Kamhi, A., Pollock, K., & Harris, J. (1996). *Communication development and disorders in African American children.* Baltimore, MD: Paul H. Brookes.

Kappa Delta Pi. (1994). *Insights on Diversity.* West Lafayette, IN: Author

Kayser, H. (1995). *Bilingual speech-language pathology.* San Diego, CA: Singular.

Kayser, H. (2002). Bilingual language development and language disorders. In D. Battle (Ed.), *Communication disorders in multicultural populations* (3rd ed., pp. 205–232). Newton, MA: Butterworth-Heinemann.

Kindler, A. (2002). *Survey of the states' limited English proficient students and available educational programs and services, 2000–2001 summary report.* Washington, DC: National Clearinghouse for English Language Acquisition & Language Instruction Educational Programs.

Krashen, S. D. (1981). *Second language acquisition and second language learning.* New York: Pergamon Press.

Krashen, S. (1992). Bilingual education and second language acquisition theory. In C. Leyba (Ed.), *Schooling and language minority students: A theoretical framework.* Los Angeles, CA: California State University Press.

Kritikos, E. P. (2003, February). Speech-language pathologists' beliefs about language assessment of bilingual/bicultural individuals. *American Journal of Speech-Language Pathology, 12,* 73–91.

Ladson-Billings, G. (2001). *Crossing over to Canaan: The journey of new teachers in diverse classrooms.* San Francisco: Jossey-Bass.

Langdon, H. W., & Cheng, L. (Eds.). (1992). *Hispanic children and adults with communication disorders: Assessment and intervention.* Gaithersburg, MD: Aspen.

Lynch, E. W., & Hanson, M. J. (1998). *Developing cross-cultural competence: A guide for working with young children and their families* (2nd ed.). Baltimore, MD: Paul H. Brookes.

McCarthy S. J. (1997). Connecting home and school literacy practices in classrooms with diverse populations. *Journal of Literacy Research, 29,* 145–182.

McLoyd, V. C. (1998). Socioeconomic disadvantage and child development. *American Psychologist, 3,* 185–204.

Molesky, J. (1988). Understanding the American linguistic mosaic: A historical overview of language maintenance and language shift. In S. L. McKay & S. C. Wong (Eds.), *Language diversity: Problem or resource? A social and educational perspective on language minorities in the United States* (pp. 27–68). Boston: Heinle.

Musselwhite, C. R. (1983). Pluralistic Assessment in Speech-Language Pathology. *Language, Speech, and Hearing Services in Schools. 14,* 29–37.

Naiman, N. (1974). The use of elicited imitation in second language acquisition research. *Working Papers in Bilingualism, 3,* 1–37.

National Association for the Education of Young Children. (1996). *Guidelines for preparation of early childhood professionals: Guidelines developed by the National Association for the Education of Young Children, Division for Early Childhood of the Council for Exceptional Children & National Board for Professional Teaching Standards.* Washington, DC: Author.

National Council for Accreditation of Teacher Education. (1994). *Approved curriculum guidelines.* Washington, DC: Author.

National Research Council, Division of Behavioral and Social Sciences and Education. (2002). *Minority students in special and gifted education.* Washington, DC: National Research Council.

Nieto, S. (2000). Affirming diversity: The sociopolitical context of multicultural education (3rd ed.). Reading, MA: Longman.

Ogbu, J. U. (1982). Cultural discontinuities and schooling. *Anthropology and Education Quarterly, 13*(4), 390–397.

Ogbu, J. U. (1992). Adaptation to minority status and impact on school success. *Theory into Practice, 31,* 287–295.

Ogbu, J. U., & Simons, H. D. (1998). Voluntary and involuntary minorities: A cultural-ecological theory of school performance with some implications for education. *Anthropology and Education Quarterly, 29,* 155–188.

Ortiz, A. (2001). English language learners with special needs: Effective instructional strategies. Center for Applied Linguistics. Retrieved October 26, 2004, from http://www.cal.org/resources/digest/0108ortiz.html

Ortiz, A. (2002). Prevention of school failure and early intervention for English language learners. In A. J. Artiles & A. A. Ortiz (Eds.), *English language learners with special education needs: Identification assessment, and instruction.* McHenry, IL: Delta Systems.

Padolsky, D. (2002, December). *How has the English language learner (ELL) student population changed in recent years?* Retrieved October 26, 2004, from National Clearinghouse for English Language Acquisition & Language Instruction Educational Programs website: http://www.ncela.gwu.edu

Pate, G. (1992). Reducing prejudice in society: The role of schools. In C. Diaz (Ed.), *Multicultural education for the 21st century* (pp. 137–149). Washington, DC: National Education Association.

Payne, Rubi. (2001). *Framework for Understanding Poverty.* RFT Publishing Co.

Peterson, P. L., & Barnes, C. (1996). Learning together: The challenge of mathematics, equity and leadership. *Phi Delta Kappan, 77,* 485–491.

Phillips, C. B. (1993). *Early childhood reform: Innovative approaches to cultural and racial diversity among families.* Alexandria, VA: National Association of State Boards of Education.

Phillips, D., & Crowell, N. A. (1994). Cultural diversity and early education: Report of a workshop. Retrieved October 24, 2004, from http://www.nap.edu

Politzer, R., & Ramirez, A. (1974). An error analysis of the spoken English of Mexican-American pupils in a bilingual school and a monolingual school. *Language Learning, 23*(1), 39–51.

Quinn, R. (1995). Early intervention: ¿Que quiere decir eso? . . . What does that mean? In H. Kayser (Ed.), *Bilingual speech-language pathology* (pp. 75–94). San Diego, CA: Singular.

Ramirez, M., & Casteneda, A. (1974). *Cultural democracy, bicognitive development and education.* New York: Academic Press.

Richard, M. A., & Emener, W. G. (2003). *I'm a people person: A guide to human service professions.* Springfield, IL: Charles C Thomas.

Richards, H. V., Brown, A., & Forde, T. (2004). *Addressing diversity in schools: Culturally responsive pedagogy.* Retrieved January 4, 2005, from U.S. Department of Education Office of Special Education Culturally Responsive Practices, Early Intervention, Literacy, and Programs website: http://www.nccrest.org

Rosa-Lugo, L. I., & Fradd, S. H. (2000). Preparing professionals to serve English-language learners with communication disorders. *Communication Disorders Quarterly, 22*(1), 29–42.

Roseberry-McKibben, C. (2002). *Multicultural student with special language needs* (2nd ed.). Oceanside, CA: Academic Communication Associates.

Roseberry-McKibben, C. (2003). *Assessment of bilingual learners: Language difference or disorders.* ASHA self-study guide. Rockville, MD: American Speech-Language-Hearing Association.

Roseberry-McKibben, C. A., & Eicholtz, G. E. (1994). Serving children with limited English proficiency in the schools:

A national survey. *Language, Speech, and Hearing Services in Schools, 25*(3), 156–164.

Rosenthal, R., & Jacobson, L. (1968). *Pygmalion in the classroom: Teacher expectations and pupils' intellectual development.* New York: Holt, Rinehart, Winston.

Schiff-Myers, N. (1992). Considering arrested language development and language loss in the assessment of second language learners. *Language, Speech, and Hearing Services in the Schools, 23,* 28–33.

Selinker, L. (1972). *Interlanguage.* IRAL, X/3, 31–53.

Seymour, H. N., Bland-Stewart, L., & Green, L. J. (1998). Difference versus deficit in child African American English. *Language, Speech, and Hearing Services in Schools, 29,* 96–108.

Seymour, H. N., Roeper, T, & deVilliers, J. (2003). Diagnostic Evaluation of Language Variation. San Antonio, TX: Psychological Corporation.

Sleeter, C. E. (1993). How white teachers construct race. In C. McCarthy & W. Crichlow (Eds.), *Race, identify and representation in education* (pp. 157–171). New York: Routledge.

Smith, M. A., Plawecki, H. M., Houser, B., Carr, J., & Plawecki, J. (1991). Age and health perceptions among elderly Blacks. *Journal of Gerontological Nursing, 17,* 13–19.

Soto, L. D. (1993). Native language school success. *Bilingual Research Journal, 17*(1 & 2), 83–97.

Spindler, G. (1987). Why have minority groups in North America been disadvantaged by their schools? In G. Spindler, (Ed), *Education and cultural process: Anthropological approaches.* Prospect Heights, IL: Waveland Press.

Stockman, I. J. (1996). The promises and pitfalls of language sample analysis as an assessment tool for linguistic minority children. *Language, Speech, and Hearing Services in Schools, 27*(4), 355–366.

Swisher, K. (1993). Learning styles: Implications for teachers. In C. Diaz (Ed.), *Multicultural education for the 21st century* (Chapter 5). Washington, DC: National Education Association of the United States.

Taylor, O., & Payne, K. (1983). Culturally valid testing: A proactive approach. *Topics in Language Disorders, 3,* 8–20.

Terrell, S. L., & Jackson, R. S. (2002). African Americans in the Americas. In D. Battle (Ed.), *Communication disorders in multicultural populations* (3rd ed., pp. 33–70). Newton, MA: Butterworth-Heinemann.

U.S. Bureau of the Census. (2000). Projections of populations by sex, race, and Hispanic origin, divisions and States: 1993–2020. Series A. 1990. Washington DC: U.S. Department of Health and Human Services. Retrieved October 26, 2004, from http://factfinder.census.gov/jsp/saff/SAFFInfo.jsp?_pageId=tp9_race_ethnicity

U.S. Department of Education Office of Special Education and Rehabilitative Services. (2002). *A new era: Revitalizing special education for children and their families.* Washington, DC: Author. Report also available at http://www.ed.gov/inits/commissionsboards/whspecialeducation/

Valdés, G., & Figueroa, R. A. (1996). *Bilingualism and testing: A special case of bias.* Norwood, NJ: Ablex.

Valli, L. (1995). The dilemma of race: Learning to be color blind and color conscious. *Journal of Teacher Education, 46*(2), 120–129.

Vygotsky, L. (1962). *Thought and language.* Cambridge, MA: Massachusetts Institute of Technology Press. (Original work published 1934.)

Washington, J. A., & Craig, H. K. (1992). Performance of low-income, African-American preschool and kindergarten children on the Peabody Picture Vocabulary Test-Revised. *Language, Speech, and Hearing Services in Schools, 23,* 329–333.

Washington, J. A., & Craig, H. K. (1999). Performances of at-risk, African American preschoolers on the Peabody Picture Vocabulary Test-III. *Language, Speech and Hearing Services in the Schools, 30,* 75–82.

Welch, M. (1998). *Enhancing awareness and improving cultural competence in health care: A partnership guide for teaching diversity and cross-cultural concepts in health professions training.* San Francisco: University of California Press.

Winfield, L. (1986). Teacher beliefs toward at-risk students in inner urban schools. *Urban Review, 4,* 253–267.

Witkin, H. A. (1967). A cognitive style approach to cross-cultural research. *International Journal of Psychology, 2,* 233–250.

Wolf, K. E. (1999). Preparing for evidence-based speech-language pathology and audiology. *Texas Journal of Audiology and Speech Pathology, 23,* 69–74.

Wolf, K. E. (2000). *Managing the Impact of Market-Driven changes in communication sciences and disorders: The health care setting.* Retrieved October 21, 2004, from http://www.capcsd.org/proceedings/2000/00_wolf.html

Wolf, K. E., & Calderón, J. L. (1999). Cultural competence: The underpinning of quality health care and educational services. *CSHA, 28*(2), 4–6. Retrieved October 20, 2004, from http://factfinder.census.gov/jsp/saff/SAFFInfo.jsp?_pageId=tp9_race_ethnicity

Zanger, V. V. (1994). "Not joined in": The social context of English literacy development for Hispanic youth. In B. M. Ferdman, R. M. Weber, & A. G. Ramirez (Eds.), *Literacy across languages and cultures* (pp. 171–198). Albany: State University of New York Press.

Zentella, A. C. (1997). *Growing up bilingual: Puerto Rican children in New York.* Malden, MA: Blackwell.

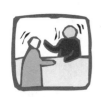

PART **III**

Where Expertise Develops

INTRODUCTION

Part III includes six chapters related to the development of expertise within a variety of practice settings. These settings include private practice, schools, nursing homes/rehabilitation facilities, hospitals, and university programs. Each chapter offers specific information related to clinical roles, funding/ reimbursement issues, clinical populations served, and the necessary support systems for moving from novice to expert. Also, these chapters allow for the comparison of various work settings. The final chapter offers the reader words of wisdom for implementing the use of information learned in this book and assists in the journey from novice to expert.

CHAPTER 10

Speech-Language Pathology in Private Practice

Nancy Swigert

> **Private Practice** A management design for a business venture that, in this textbook's context, provides services for those with speech-language-hearing problems. Such a practice may also be affiliated with or include health-care professionals from related disciplines.

 INTRODUCTION

Success in a private practice setting requires multiple aspects of knowledge, ability, and activity. This context appeals to the independent speech-language pathology practitioner who is comfortable managing a business as well as pursuing clinical expertise. In private practice, clinicians can specialize in one or more facets of the discipline, which often appeals to those who are community oriented as well as knowledgeable and skilled in marketing.

Describing the private practice setting is a daunting challenge. Private practice incorporates essential elements of practice in virtually all other settings. Private practices are broadly varied and diverse. The term *private practice* refers to the management design of a business venture. Private practices may be organized as any of the following:

- *Sole proprietorship:* One person is both owner/manager and clinician.
- *Group practice:* A clinician-owner/manager employs one or more clinicians.
- *Limited or full partnership:* All parties participate in managing the business as well as furnishing professional services.
- *Corporation:* A legal entity serves as a management umbrella for the service/business.

Private practice professional staff may include one or many specialists from one or more disciplines. The most common associations between disciplines involve physical therapy and occupational therapy, but may include counseling as well as clinical social work, clinical psychology, or psychiatry. In addition, the practice may employ licensed assistants and office support staff of one to several trained clerks, receptionists, and/or secretaries. The American Speech-Language-Hearing Association (ASHA) has defined private practice in the following way:

> A private practice is one in which a speech-language pathologist and/or audiologist, singly or in affiliation with one or more individuals
>
> **1.** Has total ethical, professional, and administrative control of the practice.
> **2.** Has total financial and legal responsibility and liability for the practice.

3. Is self-employed; that is, not an employee of an individual, organization, agency, or other entity. (This condition will be met if the practitioner is an officer of the Board of the entity and holds as much voting power as any other member of the Board, even though the practitioner may not hold stock in the entity.)
4. Accepts referrals from multiple sources and these referrals may include those obtained through independent contractor arrangements. (ASHA, 1987)

SPECIALIZATION AND DIVERSIFICATION WITHIN A PRIVATE PRACTICE

In a sole proprietor private practice, a speech-language pathologist provides services to a given population and also manages the business's marketing, fiscal responsibilities, and community relations. Services may focus on a narrow and well-defined population, for example, children ages birth to three and in a clinical setting only. Other solo practitioners might serve only corporate clients who seek to improve their presentation and oral communication skills or children and adults who stutter. One of the most rewarding features of private practice is the opportunity for working in or developing a practice that reflects the interests and specializations of the owner(s) and employees.

Not all private practices limit themselves to narrowly defined populations. Some, to ensure sufficient income to maintain and develop the business, serve clients with various disorders and from various community settings. Such a sole proprietor might see a working-age adult with a voice disorder, school-age children with language disorders, and a preschooler with a swallowing problem all in the same day. In these practices, the variety and diversity of clients/patients sustain the clinician's interest and professional development.

Many private practices that begin as solo practices grow into group practices that employ other speech-language pathologists. Within such a group practice, the speech-language pathologists might develop individual or collective expertise for specific populations, or they might all continue to see a range of clients. In accordance with the ASHA code of ethics, the private practitioner is free to establish the scope of clinical practice with the preferred clinical population(s). This flexibility and opportunity to specialize or diversify the practice of the profession appeal to many speech-language pathologists.

ROLES AND RESPONSIBILITIES IN PRIVATE PRACTICE

Private practitioners may serve literally all populations seen in other clinical settings. In addition, in a solo private practice, the professional must function in multiple capacities. The ASHA Ad Hoc Committee on Business Practices for Speech-Language Pathologists in Health Care Settings has described a continuum of knowledge and skill development for organizational managers and leaders (see Table 10.1). Many of these roles and responsibilities apply to those in private practice settings as well.

Primary roles found specifically within health-care settings (see Chapter 12 and Chapter 13 for additional information) often overlap with tasks necessary for a successful private practice.

Marketing

Tasks critical to the private practitioner in speech-language pathology include identifying and enlisting clients. Current clients also serve as "repeat resources" from which to draw new clients.

Reaching prospective clients requires specific skills. Marketing and negotiation for services are never-ending components of private practice. It is well recognized that

TABLE 10.1   Roles and Responsibilities of Speech-Language Pathologists Working in Health-Care Settings

Role	Required Knowledge	Required Skills
Leadership	Vision, communication, motivation Obtain information Understand diversity in an organization	Communicate and implement a vision Effective Interpersonal skills Awareness of and responsiveness to cultural diversity
Performance Improvement	Performance standards set by certifying/credentialing agencies Outcome measures National Outcomes Measurement system (NOMS) Benchmarking Evidence-based practice	Select and use appropriate outcome measurement tools Apply outcome data Select appropriate performance improvement measures Implement performance improvement methods.
Compliance and Professional Practice	Knowledge of regulations Facility and corporate policies Compliance rules Privacy protection Risk management Due process (ASHA code of ethics)	Implement regulations Ensure compliance with regulations Prepare policies and procedures Comply with current legislation affecting practice Comply with facility risk management Follow due process
Personnel Management	Determine appropriate staffing levels Develop competency requirements for staff Determine methods of supervision Clinical advancement Appropriate human resources (e.g., Family Medical Leave Act)	Monitor staffing Determine qualifications needed Provide opportunities for discussion of goals/problems/ideas Develop personnel policies Ensure licensure renewals Support professional development and continuing education Maintain safe environment Recruit and retain a diverse staff
Advocacy	Legislative and regulatory processes Role of lobbying Role of speech-language-hearing associations Federal, state, and local legislative processes Issues that affect organization, profession, and consumers	Educate, organize, and mobilize staff Gather data on outcomes, costs, benefits from multiple sources Effectively communicate and negotiate
Marketing	Definitions of marketing, sales, and promotion Consumer and market analysis External and internal activities to promote speech-language-hearing Customer service	Deliver products and services that satisfy customers Develop market strategies Engage in internal and external educational strategies Resolve customer complaints
Accounting/ Fiscal Management	Organization's budget process Creation of budget Accounting basics Cash-flow and balancing of budget Reimbursement Contract negotiation Technology relating to accounting processes	Plan and create budgets Analyze key accounting metrics Price services competitively Conduct cost-benefit analysis Develop fiscally relevant management tools Develop and manage contracts

Source: Modified from American Speech-Language-Hearing Association. (2004b). Knowledge and skills in business practices for speech-language pathologists who are managers and leaders in health care organizations. *ASHA Supplement 24.*

treatment outcomes are the best marketing tools the clinician possesses. The reputation of the practice benefits when clients improve, feel positive about the services they receive, and share these outcomes with others in the community. In fact, treatment outcomes readily recognized and appreciated by community networks of collaborating professionals are by far the strongest marketing tool of the private practitioner. The successful practitioner is conscientious in promoting positive outcomes for clients and the practice. Often, this means coping with constraints outside the practitioner's control. Client/patient outcomes in private practices may be influenced by limitations imposed by supporting agencies that fund these services. Outcomes reflect agency policies that dictate reimbursement limitations. Ethical practice and conscientious competition in the market for diagnosis and treatment of communication disorders within a given community distinguish the expert private practitioner (ASHA, 2004a).

A private practice can utilize many other marketing strategies to keep the community informed about the practice and the professionals working within the practice. The practice might host consumer meetings (e.g., support groups, an educational presentation for parents). Announcements may be placed in the community paper or letters may be sent directly to referral sources. Participation in community health screenings and charitable activities are other avenues for exposure and recognition.

Contracting

In addition to traditional referrals from physicians, teachers, other health-care providers, and satisfied clients, private practitioners may negotiate contracts with institutions to provide needed services. For example, diagnostic and therapeutic services may be provided in a preschool/day care, skilled nursing facility, public or private school, acute care unit, rehabilitation hospital, or in patients' homes through contractual agreement with the private practitioner. Other work sites for speech-language pathologists may include detention centers for adjudicated children or federal or state prisons. To do this successfully within economic constraints for sustaining the practice, the speech-language pathologist must negotiate a reasonable contract—a legal document of agreement—with each facility/agency.

Client/patient outcomes in private practice reflect the setting in which those services are provided. If the practice has a contractual agreement with an agency or facility, outcomes will definitely reflect reimbursement limitations as well as policies of the contracting institution.

Consider patients at various points in the **continuum of care.** Patients in an acute care facility are typically hospitalized in that unit for a short time. The services provided may be largely diagnostic and an appropriate outcome might be accurate diagnosis and education of the family to establish a basic communication system or diet modifications to allow the patient to eat safely. In the home-health setting, a successful outcome might be ensuring that each individual who shares the patient's home can communicate with the patient during daily living activities. The patient must be considered "homebound" to qualify for services of a home-health agency. Thus, as the patient's ability to be ambulatory and reintegrate within a social context improves, he or she may no longer qualify for services. The outcome may be affected by the length of time the patient is funded for home-health agency services. Certainly, the traits, knowledge, and skills essential to expertise are critical to negotiate the contracts for these types of populations (ASHA, 2004b).

Business Management

Most private practices must carefully monitor cash flow to meet tight budgets or narrow operating margins. If extra or unbudgeted income becomes available, it may be designated for professional travel expenses or for continuing education course fees. Because private practices stand alone, they cannot count on multiple monetary resources as larger institutions such as hospitals or freestanding clinics may provide.

Typical expenses may include rent, lease, or purchase payments for office space, professional equipment, supplies, tests, and materials; professional fees and dues; staff salary(s); business management consultant fees; insurance, utilities, phone, and janitorial service costs. If diagnostic and therapy services fail to generate sufficient income, the private practitioner must be prepared to approach financial institutions (banks, loan corporations) for credit assistance and to compete in the community for contractual opportunities (ASHA, 2004b).

Documentation

Every setting benefits from having a tool to measure outcomes and a benchmark against which to compare those outcomes. ASHA provides the **National Outcomes Measurement System (NOMS)** for use with pre-kindergarten children and another for adults. (See Chapter 12 for a more thorough discussion of NOMS.) The NOMS can be an especially useful tool for private practices as it affords credibility to their reported outcome measures. That is, instead of private practice personnel merely describing client outcomes, they can also state how their outcomes compare to a national norm. The private practice clinician is responsible for using evidence-based practice. (See Chapter 7 for additional information.) This means that he or she chooses only evaluation and treatment regimens backed up by solid scientific evidence to show that they are efficacious. **Efficacious treatment** is effective and efficient treatment that obtains the desired effects. Compare this to **treatment outcome,** which describes the results of typical care delivered in a typical way, without any "research" controls. In clinical settings, when we say *efficacy,* we typically refer to outcomes. Novice clinicians may need guidance in analyzing data related to techniques to determine if the evidence is sound. Whether novice or experienced, the clinician must carefully select the techniques and procedures to be used with the client and inform the client when using experimental procedures.

ASHA's Research and Scientific Affairs Committee has provided an excellent summary for the need to conduct evidence-based practice in communication disorders. This report discusses explicit criteria against which to evaluate the quality of evidence to support our clinical decisions. The authors identify five themes to address in evidence ratings:

- *Independent confirmation and converging evidence* usually obtained from multiple sources and even meta-analysis of many independently conducted clinical studies.
- *Experimental controls* obtained from development of controlled experiments that place one group of participants in a controlled group and another group in an experimental group are generally more respected than are retrospective clinical-records studies.
- *Avoidance of subjectivity and bias* usually takes place in using controlled blinds, concealment, and masking of patient assignment to groups or treatments protocols.
- *Effect size and confidence intervals* should be included in each clinical study reviewed for evidence-based practice and selection of treatment effects.
- *Relevance and feasibility* is particularly important to the study of patients most commonly seen within the specific clinical practice (ASHA, 2004c).

Although private practitioners may lack sufficiently large caseloads to directly participate in evidence-based research, they can certainly read relevant literature and draw conclusions for their practice based on the accumulating literature. For example, literature is increasing in adult practice of neurogenic disorders (Robey, 1998; Yorkston et al., 2001a, b) as is literature related to services provided for children (Casby, 2001; Helfand et al., 2001).

Billing and Payment of Fees

Some clients of private practices pay for their services "out of pocket." This may be because the practice has chosen not to participate in insurance plans, because the disorder is not covered by insurance, or because the client chooses to continue services after insurance has discontinued reimbursement for services. If the patient receives services in an outpatient setting through contractual arrangement and wants to use insurance to pay for the services, then the outcome will reflect the amount of service for which the payer is willing to reimburse. Many insurance companies do not cover diagnosis or treatment for speech-language disorders, especially if the patient's age leads them to consider the problem the school system's responsibility and covered by federal, state, and local funding sources. Some may cover a limited number of visits if the communication disorder is related to a medical condition (such as hoarse voice due to vocal nodules). For example, a managed-care company might pay for eight therapy sessions for a voice disorder. Thus, the predicted outcome for that patient (the **prognosis**) must take into account what can be accomplished within the restricted amount of time. The private practitioner must be familiar with all payment options available to clients/patients; federal, state, and community resources; and the methods for billing for reimbursement. Often, a knowledgeable and experienced staff member handles filing appropriate documentation required for reimbursement.

Developing the Practice

Private practices may hire speech-language pathologists in their clinical fellowship year. However, the candidate must give evidence of a strong graduate school academic and clinical record. The small or beginning private practice may lack the advantage of a recognized "institutional name" in the community (e.g., the University Speech and Hearing Clinic, the Community Hospital Department, a large well-established private practice). Each member of the practice, including the clinical fellow, must add value and recognition.

An experienced clinician mentors and supervises the clinical fellow. Also, the novice can observe more experienced clinicians as they provide services and can participate in continuing education. The novice clinician soon discovers that learning did not end with graduation. Instead, the novice must seek out every opportunity to read, observe, study, discuss, and continue to learn.

Many practices also employ speech-language pathology assistants as support personnel. The assistant's role often is defined and regulated by state agencies, as well as professional organizations. Guidelines for employing, training, and supervising speech-language pathology assistants are available through state licensing agencies and the ASHA Task Force on Support Personnel (ASHA, 2004c). These important guidelines help protect clients/patients and assistants by outlining the roles and responsibilities of the supervisor and the assistant.

Professional Development

Private practitioners are often on the forefront of advances in the profession and thus often venture into new areas of practice on the cutting edge. Because they are not bound by cumbersome institutional policies and procedures, private practitioners can more readily assume reasonable risks and enter these new areas. Risk in practice necessitates wisdom in selecting and applying techniques, in research awareness, and in networking with specialists who can act as resources to help diminish risk factors.

Furthermore, ASHA's Board of Ethics stresses that members must continue professional development throughout their careers. One area of mandated knowledge is cultural competency. The ASHA code of ethics requires

> . . . the provision of services to all populations and recognition of the cultural/linguistic or life experiences of both professionals and those they serve. Everyone has a culture. Therefore, cultural competence is as important to successful provision of services as are scientific, technical, and clinical knowledge and skills. (ASHA, 2005)

New interests in services continue to arise. A recent area of practice derived from knowledge of cultural competence is corporate speech pathology. **Corporate speech pathology** services differ in that a company is the client. The company seeks these services when employees need to improve oral and written communication skills. In our increasingly multicultural society, companies may have employees for whom English is a second language. They may have accent or dialect differences that interfere with successful completion of their jobs. The services are typically provided at the work site, and often in a "class" instead of one-on-one.

Private practitioners in independent settings may have limits on the speech-language pathology services they can provide by virtue of the practice's physical setting and associated professionals. Often, these services are provided by speech-language pathologists who work in medical settings. Two examples come easily to mind, one related to voice and one to swallowing. A speech-language pathologist can use videostroboscopy to diagnose voice disorders only in a physician's office. Some speech-language pathologists in private practice contract their services to otolaryngologists to perform this procedure. Medicare mandates that use of fiber-optic endoscopy for evaluation of swallowing disorders be completed with physician supervision. This typically means that the physician is present in the same office suite. In a hospital setting, the supervision is "presumed." Therefore, speech-language pathologists in private practice who want to see clients with voice and swallowing disorders typically do so through a contractual arrangement with a physician's group or hospital (ASHA, 2001).

CLINICAL EXPERTISE IN PRIVATE PRACTICE

The private practitioner can focus on areas of preferred practice with specific clinical populations and in a variety of contexts. Additionally, the private practitioner assumes responsibility for continual marketing that sells the services to a community. If the community already has speech-language services, new private practices endeavor to offer slightly different, more extensive, or specialized service(s). If the community has no competing private practice speech-language services, the newly opening clinical business must educate the public, promote the concept of need for the services to the available population, and provide services the community needs and wants with sufficient vigor that income meets the costs of doing business.

The interests, traits, talents, abilities, and skills that provide for all of these activities reflect those presented in Chapter 3, which describes the five factors of clinical expertise: interpersonal skills, professional skills, problem-solving skills, technical skills, and knowledge and experience. Certainly considerable ability in each of these areas is critical to anyone who works successfully in a private practice setting.

Interpersonal Skills

The novice clinician in private practice expends constant energies to interact with the clientele and their caregivers as well as with other personnel. Compliance with established standards of the community and within the practice may be new or may differ from the clinician's previous environments. Keen observation and careful inquiry can be particularly appropriate for clinicians entering the treatment setting for the first time. The new clinician in a private practice setting represents that practice during each meeting with a new client, patient, or colleague. It is crucial that clinic services reflect competence, enthusiasm, and sincerity. To be a valuable member of the practice, clinicians must be flexible and willing to broaden their scope of practice or to try new ways of approaching new phenomena. For example, even if a clinician were hired to see mostly pediatric patients, the practice might need him or her to see adults.

Clinicians interested in developing expertise in the area of interpersonal skills would benefit from serving as the "front person" for the practice. That is, attending meetings for the practice owner/administrator, meeting clients, or perhaps participating in an interview for a community paper. This expertise would be highly valued in a private practice. Clinicians whose interpersonal skills allow them to help build the practice and not merely maintain it, are recognized and would likely advance in the practice.

Professional Skills

Of course, it is accepted without question that the entering private practitioner in speech-language pathology holds all required certifications and licenses and that ongoing continuing education is part of the practice routine. Another part of private practice, building public recognition of the proprietor and clinicians, may involve the clinic personnel in clinical research presented at state and national professional meetings and conferences as well as at local programs. These activities are often considered newsworthy and appear in the local newspaper or on the local electronic media. Such professional recognition can help attract new clients and encourage fellow professionals to refer patients and clients to the private practitioner. All these and other efforts to place the practice at the disposal of the public are part of marketing the practice.

Among the professional skills described in Chapter 3, one of critical significance in private practice is resource management (use without waste of available time, personnel, materials, equipment, and space). Meeting the cost of maintaining a private practice means generating sufficient income to cover incurred expenses. To succeed, the private practitioner must demonstrate skill in developing and applying a **strategic business plan** that outlines and details revenue sources, expenditures, practice growth, and other issues critical to practice success. Some practices hire a business manager or consultant to assist with developing and directing the business plan.

The **revenue** (money) that comes into the private practice typically goes right back out to pay expenses. Therefore, it is important that all members pay careful attention to managing resources and understanding various payment methods. While larger institutions may be able to write off an occasional bad debt when a client fails to pay for services, bad debts can put a private practice out of business. The ability to identify and approach new sources of business with a thoroughly thought-out plan of service offerings also falls under this factor. The private practitioner who is creative and aware of community attitudes, goals, and needs can design branches of the business venture to satisfy those needs and earn recognition for forwarding the larger more inclusive efforts to achieve selected goals.

The clinician who can independently manage the caseload, is willing to take on any client assigned, and knows how to evaluate and plan treatment demonstrates professional skills expertise. If he or she lacks a sufficient knowledge base regarding treatment of a specific disorder area, the clinician seeks consultation with other colleagues to access the information. Such professionals complete detailed records in a timely manner and in a meaningful format for review as needed by other professionals. The supervisor never has to worry about checking that clinician's charts. The clinician developing expertise ensures that no services are provided until necessary **preauthorization** (pre-approval of services) is in hand and all documentation requirements are met. Expertise may be acknowledged by assigning a clinician to mentor and supervise others.

Problem-Solving Skills

Beginning clinicians need to recognize that every decision they make reflects not only their own problem-solving skills but also affects practice integrity. In the business of a private practice, practitioners must approach problems with confidence and comfort. The clinician must show careful attention to detail, be thorough, and follow through on decisions. The skilled clinician knows when to request assistance from a colleague or from outside sources, as well as when to make a responsible referral. With today's conflicting policies in health-care delivery administration, those who choose to receive services at a private practice setting expect service quality above and beyond what they might receive in an institutional setting.

The expert clinician demonstrates superior problem-solving skills. These skills are reflected in the ability to manage a caseload independently and ensure maximum productivity for time expended. In any setting, time is money. In a private practice, this is even more apparent. Time management expertise that increases revenue for the practice is typically recognized through monetary rewards. The practice owner generally makes every effort to retain such a clinician. The expert clinician also begins to see the "big picture" for the practice. That is, the clinician's concern extends beyond the clinical caseload to the practice's health and reputation and he or she actively explores ways to improve each.

Technical Skills

The technical skills needed to work in a private practice do not differ significantly from skills needed in any other speech-language pathology work setting. However, as mentioned, clients who choose to receive treatment in a private practice expect the best available service. This includes seeing professionals whose technical skills eliminate error and doubt regarding treatment benefits and outcomes.

Expertise in technical skills is recognized in private practice much as it is in other settings. The technical expert often is assigned the most challenging clinical clients or becomes a mentor for newer clinicians. Expertise in technical skills may indeed correlate with better outcomes for clients. In addition, the desired outcome may be achieved in a more efficient way.

Knowledge and Experience

The knowledge and experience needed to begin clinical work in a private practice are similar to those needed in any clinical setting. Because private practice clinicians may work quite independently, they must be active and dedicated lifelong learners. Practices value most the new colleagues (and employees) who took initiative as students in seeking practicum experiences in various types and severities of disorders and different clinical settings.

Knowledge and experience continues to be an area of growth recognized by practice owners. The most valuable practice members are those who continually seek to increase their knowledge. They seek out opportunities for continuing education, whether attending a conference or reading an article. They do not wait for the owner to identify their needs for improvement. They recognize these independently and search for ways to enhance their knowledge base. This initiative is recognized and the employee may be afforded the opportunity to attend a conference or workshop.

RECOGNITION OF EXPERTISE

The clinician in private practice looks for every opportunity to demonstrate expertise to those who refer clients for services. One of the best ways to do this is through sharing reports, treatment plans, and other documentation with referral sources. Each time a physician, for example, receives an accurate, clear, and concise report from the practice, the physician is likely to remember the practice the next time a patient needs referral for speech-language services.

Private practitioners recognize expertise developing in an employee in different ways. The employee may have success with a particularly challenging client or clients may start to ask for a clinician by name (e.g., "My neighbor saw that clinician, and I would like my child to see her, too"). These indicators of recognizable levels of consumer preference are the beginnings of expertise.

Private practices are often less formal in their management, including promotions, than larger institutions may be. A private practice, for example, may not have a published **organizational chart** that identifies the "chain of command" and position/job descriptions, or even an approved budget. Position titles such as department manager, director, or assistant vice president are less likely. A sizable practice might have divided supervisory or managerial duties among the employees but might not assign specific titles or even devise detailed job descriptions. Less-structured settings have both advantages and disadvantages. The practice may offer employees more flexibility in hours worked, days worked, time off. On the other hand, a less clearly defined career ladder may leave employees with less information about opportunities for advancement and methods of recognition.

Another way that private practices recognize expertise is by delegating more responsibility. For example, a practice member may move into a new role, such as coordinating new referrals or meeting with prospective corporate clients. The clinician developing technical expertise may be encouraged to be more selective in the types of clients accepted. For example, a clinician who was initially expected to see all types of clients may begin to develop a real expertise in dealing with adults with voice disorders. As a result, the clinician might request a caseload that allows specialization and the opportunity to see all voice patients referred to the practice.

The practice might recognize expertise by branching out into a new area. This might include purchasing specialized tests or equipment or marketing the new area aggressively. Perhaps one of the clinicians develops expertise in social communication disorders. The practice might invest in new tests related to the area and mount a marketing campaign to let area schools and physicians know that this clinician can expertly serve these clients.

Expertise can also bring financial recognition and reward. How this is done will depend on how the practice is structured. Some private practices treat their employees as salaried staff and provide benefits. Some practices offer bonuses to clinicians who generate a certain amount of revenue for the practice. Some practices pay their employees a percent of the revenue they generate.

Recognition within the private practice may come in subtle ways. The owner may seek the clinician's input in making decisions about the future of the practice. These may be small decisions (e.g., what test the practice should purchase) to big decisions (e.g., should we pursue a contract with a new agency). The clinician may be recognized at a staff meeting or may find that the owner suggests that other employees seek out the clinician's opinion. Recognition may be as simple as being asked to stay on with the practice and continue to help it grow.

Accountability

It is a challenge to quantify the relationship between a clinician's level of expertise and client outcome, but subjectively it is thought to exist. The experienced clinician does *not* waste time in treatment sessions trying methods not proven effective. The experienced clinician has tried different methods with different clients, has reviewed evidence-based practice research, and has knowledge of the most effective treatment methods.

The experienced clinician has had successes and failures and has learned from both—probably more from the failures than from the successes. This relates to intuitive/tacit knowledge. Consider an example from voice therapy and one from swallowing therapy. The novice voice clinician might spend several sessions discussing with the adult client how she feels when her voice breaks when she is trying to teach her second-grade class. She might ask the client to describe in detail the children's reactions to the voice breaks. The experienced clinician provides immediate suggestions for changing the teacher's vocal patterns and perhaps for modifying the classroom environment in which she is teaching. While the novice clinician is spending time discussing the teacher's feelings, the experienced clinician is using the few therapy sessions the insurance company has approved to make practical changes in the teacher's vocal use.

The novice clinician may designate that a patient eat nothing by mouth (NPO) when seeing a little penetration of liquids into the upper laryngeal vestibule on the modified barium swallow. The experienced clinician knows from reading the literature and from experience with many other diagnostic studies personally performed, that penetration of thin liquids can be entirely within normal limits. The novice clinician might unduly restrict the patient's intake through lack of knowledge and experience.

SUMMARY

A private practice in speech-language pathology is a business enterprise and can be an exciting and challenging setting in which to work. New clinicians often have more responsibility and more flexibility within both the clinical suites and business offices than they might find within a larger institution. Clinicians generally have choices of becoming involved in many aspects of the profession and its practice rather than total emersion in client care. Private practice can be the ideal setting in which to demonstrate and apply the independence of speech-language pathologists as competitive business entrepreneurs as well as incisive decision makers and case managers for clients with communication and swallowing disorders. The private practice setting provides an excellent environment for developing professional expertise.

THOUGHTS FOR EXPLORATION

1. What skills are necessary to be successful in private clinical practice?
2. What are some rewards of working in a private practice setting?
3. In a multidisciplinary private practice:
   a. What disciplines may be represented on staff?
   b. How do the different disciplines compliment each other?

REFERENCES

American Speech-Language Hearing Association. (1987, March). Private Practice. *ASHA, 29*, 35.

American Speech-Language-Hearing Association. (2001). *Scope of practice in speech-language pathology*. Rockville, MD: Author.

American Speech-Language-Hearing Association. (2004a). *Medicare Fee Schedule for Speech-Language Pathologists*. Available at http://www.ASHA.org.

American Speech-Language-Hearing Association. (2004b). Knowledge and skills in business practices for speech-language pathologists who are managers and leaders in health care organizations. *ASHA Supplement 24*.

American Speech-Language-Hearing Association. (2004c). *Guidelines for the training, use, and supervision of speech-language pathology assistants* [Guidelines]. Available at http://www.asha.org.

American Speech-Language-Hearing Association. (2005). Cultural competence. *ASHA Supplement 25*.

Casby, M. W. (2001). Otitis media and language development: A meta-analysis. *American Journal of Speech-Language Pathology, 10*, 65–80.

Helfand, M., Thompson, D., Davis, R., McPhillips, H., Lieu, T. L., & Homer, C. J. (2001 October) *Newborn hearing screening: A summary of the evidence for the U.S. Preventive Services Task Force*. Rockville, MD: Agency for Healthcare Research and Quality. Available at http://www.ahcpr.gov.

Robey, R. R. (1998). A meta-analysis of clinical outcomes in the treatment of aphasia. *Journal of Speech, Language, and Hearing Research, 41*, 172–187.

Yorkston, K. M., Spencer, K., Duffy, J., Beukelman, D., Golper, L. A., Miller, R., et al. (2001a). Evidence-based medicine and practice guidelines: Application to the field of speech-language pathology. *Journal of Medical Speech-Language Pathology, 4*, 243–256.

Yorkston, K. M., Spencer, K., Duffy, J., Beukelman, D., Golper, L. A., Miller, R., et al. (2001b). Evidence-based practice guidelines for dysarthria: Management of velopharyngeal function. *Journal of Medical Speech-Language Pathology, 4*, 257–274.

CHAPTER **11**

Speech-Language Pathology Services in the Schools

Nancy Huffman and Kathleen Whitmire

Exceptional Student Education (ESE) Educational programs that provide specially designed instruction to meet the needs of students who vary from the norm and who are eligible for special education and related services, including those who are gifted and talented as well as those with disabilities.

INTRODUCTION

In the school setting, speech-language pathologists discover perhaps the broadest array of communication disorders, delays, and needs in a single setting. School-based clinicians must maintain high skill levels in diagnosing and treating all communication disorders. Additionally, the clinical practitioner must understand and integrate practice into educationally relevant goals that help students learn and make expected academic progress. In this setting, you must become an advocate for your profession and work cooperatively in achieving both speech-language and educational outcomes.

The speech-language pathologist who chooses to practice in schools steps into an education system historically hierarchical, supported by public tax dollars, regulated by government agencies at local, state, and national levels, to help prepare children to be productive citizens. The speech-language pathologist works to create, foster, and provide an environment where students with communication disorders can achieve their potential. The school-based speech-language pathologist represents the school system in the community along with its teachers, staff, and administrators.

THE SCHOOL CONTEXT

Since their inception, school-based speech-language services have undergone profound fundamental changes in scope and focus. Social, political, and professional influences that drive these changes shape and reflect one another. Of particular relevance are issues regarding (a) the degree to which schools are held responsible for providing an education to children with disabilities, and the expectations for the nature and quality of that education; (b) our nation's changing demographics; and (c) the changing scope of speech-language pathology as a profession. True experts in school-based practice use their understanding of the role of schools within society and expectations for school-based speech-language services to make appropriate and effective clinical decisions.

Legislative/Regulatory Influences

Reauthorization of the Individuals with Disabilities Education Act (IDEA) in 1997 and again in 2004 established and provides federal funds for an educational process designed to give each student with a disability meaningful access to the general curriculum. This required speech-language pathologists to become knowledgeable about the general curriculum, that is, the same curriculum as for students without disabilities. As a result, speech-language assessments need to reflect student performance in school contexts—academic, nonacademic, and extracurricular. Speech-language goals and objectives as documented on students' individualized education programs (IEPs) must be educationally relevant and support and reflect content-area learning and student performance in various school contexts. Also, assessment and intervention depend more than ever on successful collaboration and teamwork among speech-language pathologists, special education teachers, regular education teachers, parents, and other service providers.

The No Child Left Behind Act (NCLB), the 2001 reauthorization of the Elementary and Secondary Education Act, is the principal federal law affecting education from kindergarten through high school. NCLB was designed to improve achievement for all students, including students with disabilities, English-language learners, economically disadvantaged students, and minority students. Under this act, school-based speech-language pathologists may play an important role in helping struggling students progress in regular education settings. They may consult with teachers regarding effective instructional methods or provide short-term remediation for struggling students before or instead of referring them to special education. This places a greater emphasis on speech-language pathologists' role with nondisabled students in regular education settings.

Demographic Shifts

Our nation's demographics have undergone rapid changes over the past few decades. It is now estimated that nearly one of every three citizens is African American, Hispanic, Asian American, or Native American. The limited English-proficient population is the fastest-growing population in America (ASHA, 1999). This has produced a current student population more culturally and linguistically diverse than ever before, requiring bias-free assessments and interventions.

Medical advancements have affected our nation's demographics, as well. More children survive neonatal and early childhood traumas and illnesses, although those who survive are often mentally, physically, or medically challenged. Additionally health-care reforms allow many patients to be released earlier from hospitals or rehabilitation centers; those who enter public schools often require intensive speech-language services (ASHA, 1999). School-based speech-language pathologists must be prepared to respond to these students' needs, particularly in the areas of dysphagia and assistive technology.

Professional Practice Trends

Current trends in practice are grounded in the same concepts of contextually based assessment and intervention (ASHA, 1989, 1991a, 1999, 2000a; Council for Exceptional Children, 2000; Huffman, 1992; National Joint Committee on Learning Disabilities, 1994, 1998) and increased use of collaboration and teamwork (ASHA, 1991a, 1991b, 1992, 1996, 1999, 2000a; Council for Exceptional Children, 2000; National Joint Committee on Learning Disabilities, 1991) that have emerged from the social and political changes during the past 25 years. Professional policy statements, professional consultation materials, and continuing education seminars and sessions have emphasized both skills needed and rationales for (a) assessments that go beyond standardized measures,

(b) treatment plans integrated with daily activities, and (c) a full range of service delivery options that depend on successful collaboration and teamwork with families and other professionals.

ROLES AND RESPONSIBILITIES OF THE SCHOOL-BASED SPEECH-LANGUAGE PATHOLOGIST

Most people believe a school-based speech-language pathologist primarily works directly with students with disabilities, with some time devoted to assessment and evaluation. However, the school-based speech-language pathologist assumes many roles and responsibilities in the course of the school year. Those responsibilities are outlined in Table 11.1.

In addition to direct services to students, speech-language pathologists engage in a wide range of indirect activities both with and on behalf of students. Those activities support students in their classroom activities, the general curriculum, and schoolwide activities (e.g., helping teachers match teaching style to student needs, supporting pre-referral intervention activities for nondisabled children, designing adaptations to the curriculum). Indirect activities also support students' IEP goals (e.g., participating on student planning teams, training classroom personnel to use assistive technology, planning for student transitions beyond high school). As speech-language pathologists develop expertise in school-based practice, they establish a role within the broad school community that includes contributions to districtwide activities and also become more adept at developing a work schedule that accommodates the full range of activities both with and on behalf of students (ASHA, 2002).

Literacy

Speech-language pathologists now fill an increasingly important role in literacy development as part of their expanding role in schools. Reading and writing fall within the speech-language pathologist's scope of practice (ASHA, 2001d), dyslexia has become acknowledged as a language-based learning disability (IDA, 2000), and the connections between spoken and written language are well established (ASHA, 2001e). Speech-language pathologists' knowledge of normal and disordered language acquisition, and

TABLE 11.1 Roles and Responsibilities of the School-Based Speech-Language Pathologist

- Advocacy
- Assessment/evaluation
- Caseload management
- Counseling
- Curriculum development
- Dismissal
- Documentation and accountability
- Eligibility determination
- Identification
- IEP/IFSP development
- Intervention
- Participation in school committees
- Prevention
- Reevaluation
- Research
- Supervision
- Transition
- Training and support for parents and other professionals

their clinical experience in developing individualized programs for students, prepare them to assume various roles related to reading and writing development. They fill a critical and direct role in literacy development for students with communication disorders and also aid school district or community literacy efforts on behalf of all children. These roles often include collaboration with other literacy experts (ASHA, 2001e).

Collaboration

All of the activities outlined above need collaboration and/or consultation with family members and other professionals to be effective. Collaboration is a core concept in school-based practice today. From initial identification to planning to implementation and follow-up, teams of educators and family members work together on behalf of the child (CEC, 2000). Classroom teachers can contribute to team discussions by outlining their expectations for students within their classrooms and content areas. Speech-language pathologists, special education teachers, and other related service providers, in turn, explain the challenges students with disabilities face as they attempt to meet the classroom teacher's expectations. Parents contribute information about their child's behavior and challenges outside the school setting as well as their goals and future plans for their child (CEC, 2000).

Collaboration/consultation can present challenges for even the veteran clinician and can be daunting for novices. Efforts may be hindered by risks of reduced autonomy (Nelson & Kinnucan-Welsch, 1992) and confusion regarding the roles of the classroom teacher and the speech-language pathologist (Ehren, 2000). Some speech-language pathologists express concern that collaborative intervention makes them feel like classroom teachers, aides, or tutors rather than therapists and that their therapy has become "watered down" in the classroom (Ehren, 2000). To overcome these obstacles, Ehren suggests that speech-language pathologists maintain a "therapeutic focus" while sharing the responsibility for student success. To accomplish this, speech-language pathologists should be viewed as expert in language and knowledgeable about curriculum content, whereas teachers are expert in curriculum content and knowledgeable about language. The therapeutic process is viewed as distinct from instruction in that it is more intensive and prescriptive, requiring greater expertise in the nature and development of language and language disorders. Approaching services in the schools from this perspective of "expertise plus knowledge" and the distinct expertise brought to the team by each professional can help new speech-language pathologists establish themselves within building/district teams and culture.

OUTCOMES IN THE SCHOOLS

School districts, parents, and taxpayers are interested in results. They consistently ask, "How does your service result in Manuel's ability to perform academically?" To be even more simplistic, as one administrator queried, "Tell me how what you do helps Isabella to pass reading, math, English, and social studies." School-based speech-language pathologists must be prepared to respond to these questions and produce data to support their responses.

The expert school-based speech-language pathologist selects treatment strategies and makes treatment decisions based on evidence that supports the treatment for a particular condition in a particular circumstance. Further, the speech-language pathologist must be familiar with evidence that supports various education-based instructional methods to ensure treatments not only clinically relevant but educationally relevant as well. The ASHA website http://www.asha.org is an excellent source of basic information on evidence-based practice and practice guidelines. Other sources, such as the International Reading Association website, http://www.reading.org, provide information on reading instruction based on research evidence. Dollaghan (2004), Robey (2004), and Cox (2004) provide informative discussions of application of evidence-based practice in day-to-day practice contexts.

In schools practice, we measure outcome by a student's ability to achieve IEP goals and objectives. The IEP with "speech pages" has largely given way to the integrated IEP whereby speech-language objectives link to state standards and curriculum goals. For example, in the integrated IEP, a language objective to be addressed by the speech-language pathologist may be embedded into a student's mathematics objective and related to word problems. Progress is measured at intervals identical to those of students in general education. In this example, the student's progress might be judged by teachers, the speech-language pathologist, and/or performance on standardized/nonstandardized assessments as specified by the IEP team. An articulation goal embedded in the academic area of English might look like this: "When giving oral reports, student will use age appropriate sound production with ___ % accuracy." Or a fluency goal within science may be "Student will use 75% fluent speech patterns when requesting information/asking for clarification in earth science."

Outcomes in schools practice are also measured in terms of service delivery models and length of stay in a particular service model. Consider the notion of speech-language intervention in schools as a "therapeutic" service versus an "accommodation" service. Therapeutic service implies that a specific treatment will produce a "cure" or "correction." In this context, the treatment might involve teaching a skill, providing drill and practice, or engineering opportunities for generalization. The service may be highly intensive (daily, individual treatment). Changes in student speech behavior can be tabulated and demonstrated. The service recipient usually experiences an amelioration or correction of the communication disorder. Conclusion of service (dismissal) frequently is an outcome.

On the other hand, in service oriented to "accommodation" or access to instruction, the recipient typically has a lifetime condition/disability. Service delivery focuses on analyzing the current circumstances (the classroom/instruction setting, the instructional subject, the job) and then working within the circumstances to design ways the student can function satisfactorily within those circumstances. Speech-language services may include environmental modification; modification of information presentation in the context in which the student must function; application of assistive technology, including use of augmentative and alternative communication systems; prompting strategies; and so forth. Services are delivered within the large group setting and may focus on supporting others (e.g., teachers, aides, job foreman, and other related service providers) involved in the instructional setting. As the student moves from grade to grade, from one job-training site to another, the communication demands change and accommodations are made. The service delivery model may vary and include consultation, a combination pull-out/push-in model, curriculum modification, collaborative/coteaching instructional models, etc. In summary, the overarching goal is reduced dependence and increased communication independence. Outcome indicators of this are declassification, dismissal, reduction in service frequency and intensity, and use of less-intensive service delivery models.

DEVELOPMENT OF EXPERTISE

The novice is a related services specialist, part of systemwide and building level staff—a faculty member! While putting into practice the knowledge and skills acquired during graduate school, the practitioner invests much energy into getting to know coworkers and understanding the school culture and district culture. The beginner for the first time is working with teachers, including many who are seasoned and expert at what they do. The novice sits on school-level teams, designs educationally relevant treatment programs, and negotiates a variety of service delivery models. It is critical to be viewed as a colleague with profession-specific competence who is collaborative, a team player, and supportive of a student's educational needs. The beginning school-based speech-language pathologist focuses on creating positive working relationships with colleagues and capitalizing on every opportunity to confidently demonstrate professional skills and knowledge.

The expert in the context of schools is known among staff and administrators and is active on school-based committees such as curriculum development, shared decision making, or committees planning school functions. The expert will also be known among parents—perhaps a leader of parent groups, perhaps active in parent-teacher groups. The expert has carefully and consistently over time educated parents, teachers, administrators, and school-board members about the relationship between communication skills and academic success. Further, the expert has provided ongoing information about the nature of speech-language-hearing disorders and their impact on learning.

The school-based speech-language pathologist functions in a variety of roles in the areas of prevention, identification, assessment, evaluation, eligibility determination, IEP and 504 Accommodation Plans development, service delivery program management, treatment, transition planning, dismissal, and counseling (ASHA, 1999). Table 11.2 provides selected examples of six roles and contrasts varying activities of novice and expert skills. In moving along the continuum from novice to proficient to expert, the school-based speech-language pathologist takes in work-site information and learns from it. The novice speech-language pathologist applies entry-level knowledge and skills, builds on previously learned information, broadens profession-specific knowledge, and applies it in the schools arena. Throughout the progression from novice to expert, the school-based speech-language pathologist continues to develop and refine skills in communication, personal interaction, conflict resolution, interpersonal behaviors, and professional behaviors. These skills are critical in separating the expert from the novice.

CREDENTIALS FOR SCHOOL SERVICE

The credentials of speech-language clinicians working in the schools vary according to state requirements. Possible credentials include ASHA's Certificate of Clinical Competence in Speech-Language Pathology (CCC-SLP), a state license, and a state teacher certificate.

ASHA's CCC-SLP sets the standard for entry-level requirements for the practice of that profession. Requirements for ASHA's CCC-SLP include the following:

- Graduate degree with major emphasis in communication disorders.
- Thirty-six graduate semester hours and a total of 400 practicum hours with at least 325 practicum hours obtained in a graduate program accredited by the ASHA Council for Academic Accreditation (CAA).
- A passing grade on the Praxis examination in speech-language pathology.
- Successful completion of a clinical fellowship under the supervision of an ASHA-certified speech-language pathologist.

Some states have what is known as "universal licensure." This is a state license to practice in all settings, including schools, typically issued and administered by the state's department of professional regulation. In other states, school practitioners are exempt from the state licensing law but must meet a separate set of requirements established by the state's department of education to obtain teacher certification. A few states require state licensure and teacher certification or state licensure plus education-specific coursework and examinations (ASHA, 2001f).

Requirements for state licenses are for the most part similar or equivalent to those for ASHA's CCC-SLP. In fact, some states automatically grant licensure if the applicant

TABLE 11.2   The Novice-to-Expert Continuum in School Settings

Role	The Novice/Beginner . . .	The Expert . . .
Prevention	Acquires knowledge of curriculum and state standards. Develops techniques and strategies to promote communication skills, literacy, and speech improvement.	Understands and communicates effectively where children with speech-language disorders will experience difficulty. Provides instructional modification and interventions.
Identification Member of the school or district child find team.	Develops awareness of team functions. Becomes familiar with state's eligibility criteria for services. Develops skills in data gathering. Completes child find/screening activities.	While collaborative, also advocates on behalf of students for appropriate placements and services. Demonstrates cultural competence and is sensitive to diversity. Can retrieve, sort, and organize information.
Assessment and Evaluation Is a member of evaluation team. Conducts independent assessments and evaluations.	Is familiar with collaborative strategies of assessment and planning process. Is familiar with state's eligibility criteria for services. Becomes familiar with federal and state regulations. Selects tests known to be valid and reliable. Participates in ethical decision making. Draws on range of resources as part of the evaluation. Understands the relationship of test performance to curricular concerns.	Has knowledge of test selection and administration. Is skilled at use, measuring, and interpretation of outcomes of tests, scales, and assessments. Differentiates for others communication "disorder," "delay," and "difference." Determines and explains the effect of disorder on educational progress. Adheres to and maintains scope of practice. Understands state laws and regulations and their application with respect to speech-language services.
Member of district placement committee for IDEA and/or 504 services	Becomes acquainted with members of the placement committee, identifies a person as a resource for aid in preparing reports. Applies eligibility criteria in determining need for services. Aware that decisions are a "team" responsibility. Relays decisions to committee. Aware that speech-language services support academic/school performance.	Has extensive knowledge of placement options. Effectively communicates the justification and rationale for services. Negotiates within the team for frequency and intensity of service as well as service delivery model. Maintains scope of practice within team; listens to and respects other points of view. Is skilled in advocacy, and conflict resolution. Exhibits highly developed communication skills and strong interpersonal skills. Holds trust and respect of team members, teachers, and parents.
Service provider (IEPs, 504 plans, general education literacy programs, speech improvement programs)	Understands service delivery models. Understands classroom curriculum and instruction and develops IEP. Develops evidence-based practice. Seeks needed assistance to develop behavior management. Engages in continuing education. Cooperates with IEP team for integrated services. Makes adjustments in frequency and intensity of services.	Is skilled in evidence-based practice. Confidently implements IEP and uses a variety of treatment protocols. Consistently seeks continuing education. Designs functional situations for students to successfully acquire or use specific skills. Is skilled in managing high-needs students through development and implementation of functional behavior plans. Can direct a "team" implementation. Skilled in developing an integrated IEP. Confidently communicates a long-term goal to promote independence. Applies the ASHA CODE OF ETHICS proactively (ASHA, 2003a). Confidently communicates child's needs to parents and handles difficult situations and discussions regarding student services.
Advocate	Understands that school administrators may not be informed about the profession.	Acquaints and updates administrators and teams on issues of professional management. Remains current on school issues.

holds the CCC-SLP. Teacher certification, on the other hand, varies across states in requirements for the master's degree (i.e., degree may be in a field "related to" communication disorders), clinical practicum (i.e., must include school experience), coursework (e.g., courses in pedagogy and child development), and examinations (e.g., a passing grade on a state teachers' exam).

In 36 states, an individual entering the public school system must have at least a master's degree to work as a speech-language pathologist (ASHA, 2001f). Of those 36 states, 7 require the practitioner to be state licensed or to meet requirements over and above a master's degree. Even in states that require incoming personnel to have at least a master's degree, individuals remain who entered the school system when only a bachelor's degree was required. Many states have set dates by which these people must receive a master's degree. Approximately 14 states allow bachelor's-level personnel to start work in public schools as speech-language pathologists. However, several of these states require that the individual be enrolled in a master's degree program and complete that program within a certain timeframe. A few of these states allow such individuals to work only under emergency certification or when a qualified master's-level individual cannot be located.

The Clinical Fellowship Year and the Probationary Appointment

School districts or states that require the ASHA CCC-SLP usually provide supervision for the ASHA clinical fellowship. In addition, some school districts, through a collective bargaining agreement (union negotiated), appoint a teacher mentor for first-year teachers. In the case of speech-language pathologists, the appointed mentor may be ASHA certified and therefore able to also serve as the ASHA clinical fellowship supervisor. In many instances, however, those in need of an ASHA clinical fellowship supervisor must use their own resources to secure an appropriately credentialed supervisor. Beginning school-based speech-language pathologist in certain cases might have both a school district supervisor/administrator and a profession-specific ASHA clinical fellowship supervisor who is not a school district employee. This varies from state to state and among school districts.

The clinical fellowship is an opportunity for first-year speech-language pathologists to expand and refine knowledge and skills acquired in graduate school. When workplace realities and professional ideals and expectations meet and sometimes clash, the guidance of a skilled clinical supervisor is essential. As the new professional continues to gain experience and confidence, behaviors developed with supportive supervision emerge.

Continuing Education

Continuing education is a requirement for maintaining teacher certification, a state's professional practice license for speech-language pathology, and ASHA's CCC-SLP. Between the particular credential(s) each state requires and the particular credentials a school-based speech-language pathologist voluntarily holds, he or she may need to fulfill multiple sets of requirements. Although individuals must demonstrate/document continuing education, the school district must provide the opportunity to do so. A school-based speech-language pathologist must be prepared to navigate the continuing education requirements pertaining to each of the credentials held.

LEARNING THE ROPES: PROFESSIONAL ISSUES

Novice school-based speech-language pathologists must obtain knowledge and skills in professional areas beyond clinical practice to develop expertise in school settings. Such professional issues include employee performance evaluations, ethics, unions, and school finance.

Employee Performance Evaluation

A school district's employee performance evaluation program represents the confluence of ideas from the district mission and goals, the teacher association/union, state regulatory requirements, and the local community. Performance evaluation programs for instructional staff (including speech-language pathologists) focus on improvement of instruction.

Evaluation programs in schools are broadly written recognizing that instructional staffs comprise individuals representing many areas of specific knowledge and skills. It is also the norm rather than the exception that teachers are evaluated relative to the same five factors of expertise identified and described in Chapter 3: interpersonal skills, professional skills, problem-solving skills, technical skills, and knowledge and experience (Graham, 1998, Graham & Guilford, 2000).

Table 11.3 provides an example summarizing the components of professional behavior used to evaluate a school district's instructional staff (including speech-language pathologists). If the reader substitutes "speech-language pathologist" for "professionals," it becomes clear that this evaluation model has application for our profession accommodating the values for supervision and evaluation of clinical performance to which we aspire.

Ethics and Expertise in Schools

School district administrators may have limited familiarity with codes of ethics of the various allied-health (helping) professions represented among their employees. They may be unacquainted with these employees' requirements to adhere to their professions' ethical codes. School-based speech-language pathologists have a strong role to play in educating administrators and coworkers even as they sort out for themselves the ethical challenges of the interplay of legal/regulatory requirements, workplace rules, and professional ethics.

TABLE 11.3   Components of Professional Behavior: Seven Areas of Professional Evaluation

Evaluation Area	Description of Expected Professional Behavior
Communication	Communication provides verbal and nonverbal messages openly and accurately and imparts specific knowledge and information.
Understanding/Knowledge of Field	Demonstrate proficiency in a particular discipline and in learning theory; use all available resources; have knowledge of purpose of education and awareness of range of available services.
Management of the Professional Environment	Organized and consistent; make good use of time, act independently, and use available resources.
Planning	Use planning as a process that involves long-term goals and short-range objectives; select strategies and resources for assessment methods of various learning styles.
Instructional Strategies	Understand productive ways to interact with students/clients; define objectives; provide active involvement, evaluate progress using creative and varied methods with ongoing feedback.
Interpersonal Skills	Demonstrate interpersonal skills required to interact successfully with students/clients and coworkers.
Additional Professional Behavior Components: 1. Administrative Responsibility 2. Willingness to Grow	*Administrative Responsibility* and *Willingness to Grow* are a part of daily routine 1. Administrative Responsibility: Attend meetings, keep records, contribute to positive public relations, and maintain confidentiality while being punctual, reliable, and ethical. 2. Willingness to Grow: Remain current, gain proficiency, evaluate needs and goals, and seek feedback and support.

Source: Monroe #1 Board of Cooperative Educational Services, 2003.

TABLE 11.4   Ethics and Their Relevance to School-Based Practice

Issues and Ethics Statement	Application to School-Based Practice
Cultural Competence (ASHA, 2004d)	Recognize one's own and students' cultural/linguistic backgrounds.
Clinical Practice by Certificate Holders in the Profession in Which They Are Not Certified (ASHA, 2004b)	Adhere to scopes of practice in speech-language pathology and audiology.
Confidentiality (ASHA, 2004c)	Provide safeguards and protection of records.
Prescription (ASHA, 2001c)	Independent judgment in the provision services.
Representation of Services for Insurance Reimbursement or Funding (ASHA, 2004e)	Accurately and fairly bill for services provided.
Clinical Fellowship Supervisor's Responsibilities (ASHA, 2004a)	Certified members provide early mentorship.
Drawing Cases for Private Practice from Primary Place of Employment (ASHA, 2001a)	Prohibitions, restrictions, and conflicts of interest.
Ethical Practice Inquiries: ASHA Jurisdictions (ASHA, 2001b)	Sources for enforcement of codes of ethics for professional conduct.

In daily work experience, infrequent or recurring situations may give rise to professional questions of ethics. At such times the ASHA *Code of Ethics* (ASHA, 2003a) and the ASHA *Issues in Ethics* statements (http://www.ASHA.org) become important sources of guidance in actual personal situations. Table 11.4 lists ASHA *Issues in Ethics* statements with particular relevance to practice in schools. An additional valuable resource is the ASHA publication, *Ethics and IDEA* (ASHA, 2003b), which uses scenarios to provide in-depth guidance regarding ethical issues that arise in schools and offers strategies for resolution. Furthermore, it is also important to remember that all treatment goals must have educational relevance for the child if treatment takes place in the educational setting.

Collective Bargaining Units, Unions, and Employee Associations

Beginning school-based speech-language pathologists quickly become familiar with the district decision-making system and the role of the collective bargaining unit. For example, in some school districts, the administration may be responsible for staffing and service delivery model decisions and the union for effecting decisions regarding work space and planning time. The novice employee networks with other speech-language pathologists in the district to discuss issues of concern and pathways to resolution. Among repeated concerns of school clinicians are caseload size, duties unrelated to speech-language that consume large portions of time, faculty and staff resistance to referring children for speech-language services, and failure of other faculty to participate in collaborative/consultative models of service delivery.

The novice quickly learns that speech-language pathologists are a small percentage of all the employees represented by the bargaining unit; the chances of the union expending energy on behalf of the small group are remote without a convincing case that the issue is of major importance to the education of children in the district (ASHA, 2000b).

In contrast, the speech-language pathologist with expertise in relationships with employee organizations knows the union structure and leadership and can negotiate the system to affect change. An expert can adopt a positive manner to enlighten colleagues on issues and opportunities and can enlist the support of teachers in resolving issues.

School Finance

School-based speech-language pathologists are focusing increasingly on the funding of and reimbursement for their services. Understanding where the money comes from and how one can influence funding streams involves knowledge and skills acquired by active involvement in school activities such as the budget cycle and budget preparation, school board review and annual approval of budgets by voters, specific sources and levels of revenue support for speech-language services, and district allocation of revenue to speech-language services.

School finance is a complex issue and varies markedly from district to district and state to state. At a bare minimum, it is essential to study local school finance as one develops expertise in a school system. School-based speech-language pathologists need to understand funding sources, reimbursement through Medicaid, funding allocations, budget creation and management, deadlines, expenditures, and anticipated needs. They also need to develop and refine their skills for influencing funding decisions, and identifying and taking advantage of opportunities to do so.

CAREER BUILDING AND DEVELOPMENT OF EXPERTISE IN SCHOOLS

Curriculum Vita

Documenting a career begins with the development and maintenance of a curriculum vita. The vita should include categories such as education, credentials, continuing education, presentations, membership in organizations and any positions held (offices, committee/task force memberships/chair, and term of service), awards and appointments, products developed, publications, and any other pertinent information. The curriculum vita will serve as a historical document of your achievements as your career path unfolds and changes.

Recognition

Many school districts regularly and publicly recognize outstanding employees. Employees are recognized by school boards for their contributions related to student achievements, professional achievements such as receiving an ASHA Award for Continuing Education (ACE), publications, innovative programs, or leadership in district initiatives. The experienced school-based speech-language pathologist applies well-honed communication skills to keep administrators and the district's public information officer regularly informed of activities and accomplishments.

Administrative Responsibilities

Speech-language pathologists often move into the administrative ranks in school districts and are successful administrators. Why? They have the following:

- Excellent understanding of curriculum.
- Extensive experience in people and student program management.
- Experience in negotiating school-based schedules.
- Experience in working on teams.
- Strong interpersonal skills with parents, teachers, and administrators.
- Practiced and honed conflict-resolution skills.
- Good organizational skills.
- Demonstrated ability to handle paperwork and documentation.
- Good listening and responding skills to different points of view.
- Ability to present information, interpret information, and provide counsel.
- Ability to advocate in a positive manner.

They simply have had myriad opportunities to develop and apply skills in the five areas of expertise discussed extensively throughout this book. In the context of schools, the career ladder might include administrative appointments specific in the area of speech-language pathology such as department chair or coordinator of speech-language services. In addition, administrative positions might include special education appointments such as chair of the committee on special education, director of special education, or director of support or related services. Finally, other administrative positions may be totally in the general education arena at levels such as assistant principal, principal, human resources, business manager, operations, assistant superintendent, or superintendent. State Departments of Education have typically defined administrative personnel categories that apply within the districts and intermediate education agencies in the state.

Department Experts

Speech-language departments in larger districts may support the speech-language pathologist's acquisition of specialized skill sets in areas such as auditory verbal therapy, dysphagia, apraxia, fluency, auditory processing, cued speech, or management of medically fragile students so that resident experts are available when needed. Districts frequently support continuing education training and preparation costs for development of expertise.

Mentoring and Supervision

Some states and districts may have contractually negotiated mentoring programs in which staff may apply to be mentors for new staff and are given release time and perhaps a stipend (salary increase) to do this. Thus, school-based speech-language pathologists with expertise in supervision are recognized and may be assigned not only staff mentoring duties but also ASHA clinical fellowship supervision.

The expert in supervision, because of accumulated experiences and professional wisdom, is highly respected among colleagues and administrators. The expert not only supervises clinical fellows and graduate students but may also be a sought-after resource for adjunct teaching and on-site clinical supervisor positions in local college or university programs. Often these experts lead the development of strong partnerships and collaborative relationships between local school districts and universities as the faculty there prepare students for practice in schools. The expert supervisor continues educational studies and enhances skills in supervision, leadership, and management as these areas pertain to school environments.

Additional Leadership Activities

Large speech-language departments may have opportunities for school-based speech-language pathologists to take leadership roles in developing continuing education programs; serving on department committees to develop profession-specific protocols, guidelines, and service delivery models; and other departmental and profession-specific projects.

SUMMARY

A career in a school setting can be exciting and rewarding for speech-language pathologists. School settings provide ample opportunities for growth in knowledge and skills and for developing true expertise. This journey towards expertise in a school setting presents many challenges but many rewards as well. As one develops expertise, other doors related to the profession may open with additional educational experiences. These career paths begin with obtaining and demonstrating expertise within the discipline. Additional time, energy, educational experience, and wise career choices may open other avenues of professional development. This continuous process of deriving excellence, as in all other work places, moves from a model of novice to expert with hard work and continuous learning.

THOUGHTS FOR EXPLORATION

1. What are some advantages of practicing the profession in a school context?
2. What are possible advantages of having speech-language personnel employed in administrative roles in an educational institution or system?
3. List the ways in which positive outcomes for students who receive speech-language services in schools may influence the child's academic performance.

REFERENCES

American Speech-Language-Hearing Association. (1989). Issues in determining eligibility for language intervention. *ASHA, 31,* 113–118.

American Speech-Language-Hearing Association. (1991a). A model for collaborative service delivery for students with language-learning disorders in the public schools. *ASHA Supplement, 5, 33,* 44–50.

American Speech-Language-Hearing Association. (1991b). Clinical forum: Collaborative/consultative service delivery. *Language, Speech, and Hearing Services in Schools, 22,* 147–155.

American Speech-Language-Hearing Association. (1992). Clinical forum: Implementing collaborative consultation. *Language, Speech, and Hearing Services in Schools, 23,* 365–372.

American Speech-Language-Hearing Association. (1996). Inclusive practices for children and youths with communication disorders: Position statement and technical report. *ASHA Supplement, 16, 38,* 35–44.

American Speech-Language-Hearing Association. (1999). *Guidelines for the roles and responsibilities of the school-based speech-language pathologist.* Rockville, MD: Author.

American Speech-Language-Hearing Association. (2000a). Clinical forum: Multiple perspectives for determining the roles of speech-language pathologists in inclusionary classrooms. *Language, Speech, and Hearing Services in Schools, 31,* 213–298.

American Speech-Language-Hearing Association. (2000b). *Working for change: A guide for speech-language pathologists and audiologists in schools.* Rockville, MD: Author.

American Speech-Language-Hearing Association. (2001a). Drawing cases for private practice from primary place of employment. *ASHA Supplement, 22,* 69–70.

American Speech-Language-Hearing Association. (2001b). Ethical practice inquiries: ASHA jurisdictions. *ASHA Supplement, 22,* 59–60.

American Speech-Language-Hearing Association. (2001c). Prescription. *ASHA Supplement, 22,* 59–60.

American Speech-Language-Hearing Association. (2001d). *Scope of practice in speech-language pathology.* Rockville, MD: Author.

American Speech-Language-Hearing Association. (2001e). *Roles and responsibilities of speech-language pathologists with respect to reading and writing in children and adolescents* (Position statement, Guidelines, Tech. Rep.). Rockville, MD: Author.

American Speech-Language-Hearing Association. (2001f). *State teacher requirements for audiology and speech-language pathology.* Rockville, MD: Author.

American Speech-Language-Hearing Association. (2002). *A workload analysis approach for establishing speech-language caseload standards in the schools: Guidelines.* Rockville, MD: Author.

American Speech-Language-Hearing Association. (2003a). Code of ethics (revised). *ASHA Supplement, 23,* 13–15.

American Speech-Language-Hearing Association. (2003b). *Ethics and IDEA.* Rockville, MD: Author.

American Speech-Language-Hearing Association. (2004a). Clinical fellowship supervisor's responsibilities. *ASHA Supplement, 24,* 36–38.

American Speech-Language-Hearing Association. (2004b). Clinical practice by certificate holders in the profession in which they are not certified. *ASHA Supplement, 24,* 39–40.

American Speech-Language-Hearing Association. (2004c). Confidentiality. *ASHA Supplement, 24,* 43–45.

American Speech-Language-Hearing Association. (2004d). *Cultural competence.* Available at http://www.asha.org

American Speech-Language-Hearing Association. (2004e). Representation of services for insurance reimbursement or funding. *ASHA Supplement, 24,* 51–53.

Council for Exceptional Children. (2000). *Developing educationally relevant IEPs: A technical assistance document for speech-language pathologists.* Reston, VA: Author.

Cox, R. M. (2004). Waiting for evidence-based practice for your hearing aid fittings? It's here! *Hearing Journal, 57*(8), 10–17.

Dollaghan, C. (2004). Evidence-based practice myths and realities. *ASHA Leader, 9*(7), 4–5, 12.

Ehren, B. J. (2000). Maintaining a therapeutic focus and sharing responsibility for student success: Keys to in-classroom speech-language services. *Language, Speech, and Hearing Services in Schools, 31,* 219–229.

Graham, S. V. (1998). Quality treatment indicators: A model for clinical expertise in speech-language pathology (Dissertation, University of South Florida, 1998).

Graham, S. V., & Guilford, A. M. (2000, November). *Beyond competence: Development of a model of clinical expertise.* Paper presented at the meeting of the American Speech-Language-Hearing Association, Washington, DC.

Huffman, N. P. (1992). Challenges of education reform. *ASHA, 34,* 41–44.

International Dyslexia Association. (2000, May). *Just the facts: Dyslexia basics* (Pub. 962). Baltimore: Author.

Monroe #1 Board of Cooperative Educational Services. (2003). *Agreement between the district superintendent of schools of board of cooperative education services for the first supervisory district of Monroe County and the BOCES United Professionals, NYSUT/AFT, AFL-CIO (July 1, 2003–June 30, 2005).* Fairport, NY: Author.

National Joint Committee on Learning Disabilities. (1991). Providing appropriate education for students with learning disabilities in regular education classrooms. *ASHA Supplement, 5, 33,* 15–17.

National Joint Committee on Learning Disabilities. (1994). Issues in learning disabilities: Assessment and diagnosis. In *Collective perspectives on issues affecting learning disabilities* (pp. 49–56). Austin, TX: PRO-ED.

National Joint Committee on Learning Disabilities. (1998). Operationalizing the NJCLD definition of learning disabilities for ongoing assessment in schools. In *ASHA Desk Reference* (Vol. 3, pp. 258a–258g). Rockville, MD: American Speech-Language-Hearing Association.

Nelson, N., & Kinnucan-Welsch, K. (1992). Curriculum-based collaboration: What is changing? *ASHA, 34,* 41–44.

Robey, R. R. (2004). Levels of evidence. *ASHA Leader, 9*(7), 5.

U.S. Congress. (1997). *Individuals with Disabilities Education Act Amendments of 1997.* Washington, DC: U.S. Government Printing Office.

CHAPTER 12

Speech-Language Pathology in Nursing Homes, Rehabilitation Facilities, and Community-Based Service Providers

Pete Johnson

Long-Term Care Care provided by professionals in health care and residential facilities for patients who require extended nursing or rehabilitation services.

INTRODUCTION

Nursing homes, rehabilitation settings, and community-based settings often provide long-term care and ongoing therapies. In addition to the presence of challenging communication disorders they see, these settings are undergoing major changes in service delivery directly influenced by national health-care issues. The practicing clinician must stay abreast of changing requirements for productivity, third-party payment, and funding-approved service levels. These issues influence how clinicians deliver services in these settings and reflect unique areas for development of expertise.

Nursing homes provide rehabilitation in a long-term health-care setting. Rehabilitation facilities may provide either inpatient or outpatient care. Community-based service providers encompass the widest range of settings, including home care, hospice, and specialized training centers. These three health-care settings share more similarities than differences. In every instance, they seek to reduce length and frequency of inpatient institutionalization. This is particularly true in the case of community-based service providers. The most frequently used community-based service provider is the home-care setting. Most of our discussion of community-based service providers in this chapter will focus on home health, which represents numerous employment opportunities for speech-language pathologists.

Clinical expertise in any of these settings is defined as the ability to diagnose and treat all of the common and exceptional patient diagnoses; document and code these diagnoses correctly; and utilize all treatment and non-treatment areas of practice (i.e., business knowledge, marketing, and advocacy) to effectively improve the treatment and business environment in each of the health-care settings.

The speech-language pathologist with clinical expertise understands all diagnoses related to rehabilitative care. This includes such disorders as dementia, cerebrovascular accident (CVA), closed head injury (CHI), chronic obstructive pulmonary disease (COPD), Alzheimer's disease, pneumonia, Parkinson's disease, Huntington's disease, amyotrophic lateral sclerosis (ALS), and muscular dystrophy. In addition, the speech-language pathologist with expertise presents a strong and thorough understanding of communication and swallowing disorders within these disorders. These disorders can impact communication and swallowing disorders differently, given the particular age of the patient. The speech-language pathologist with expertise working in any of the identified settings also must be well versed in the following: cervical and thoracic auscultation; analysis of lab values; patient/family interaction variables; medications influencing communication, swallowing, and behavioral variables; the effect of aging on performance; and the influence of depression and loss on patient communication and swallowing behaviors.

In addition, the speech-language pathologist with expertise can easily identify (screen), evaluate, and remediate patients with early communication and swallowing disorders before these disorders affect *functional* communication and/or swallowing ability. The speech-language pathologist with expertise also has a strong understanding of the third-party payer mechanism, and works efficiently within the reimbursement structure.

Documentation of services reflects the *treatment given* to the patient. In addition, the coding of the session best reflects the nature of the treatment modalities given to the patient. The speech-language pathologist is efficient in treatment—as well as effective. The treatment modalities are consistent with the profession's description of "best practice." The speech-language pathologist with expertise also pursues continuing education to increase therapy efficiency and effectiveness. The therapist has a thorough understanding of business practices whether employed, under contract, or an independent practitioner in any of the settings. The principles of business are an essential ingredient to functioning successfully in any health-care setting.

SPEECH-LANGUAGE PATHOLOGIST'S PROFILE

The speech-language pathologist working in a nursing home may also identify with the terms "geriatric care facility" or "long-term care facility." Speech-language pathologists working in a rehabilitation facility and/or home-care agency most likely also have a majority of geriatric patients on their caseload. Many individuals consider geriatric patients rather unchanging; however, the geriatric population (like the general population) changes on a daily basis. Their needs and problems change just as rapidly as do those of others. As a result, treatment goals may change from improving skills to regaining lost skills or developing adaptive skills. These patients rely on the speech-language pathologist to *modify treatment goals frequently to achieve functional gains in communication and swallowing activities.*

> Working within this setting can be very stimulating to the speech-language pathologist that loves the challenge of problem-solving, recognizes the benefits of interdisciplinary evaluation and planning, and appreciates the rewards of seeing a resident return to a higher level of function or stabilizing after a decline in health. (ASHA, 2004a, p. 1)

Of the three settings, the nature of nursing home practice has changed most dramatically in the past twenty years. Before 1987, most skilled-nursing facilities had few rehabilitation professionals. Speech-language pathologists in such facilities worked part time and focused on communication disorders caused by dementia. The 1987 Omnibus Budget Reconciliation Act changed the scope of practice in skilled-nursing facilities, by stating that patients needed to be brought to their *highest level of function*. In addition, the act called for a *plan* for each patient to ensure continued functioning at the highest level. All of the rehabilitation disciplines, including speech-language pathology, were then employed in the skilled-nursing facility to meet that mandate. Speech-language pathologists also began treating other disorders such as Parkinson's disease, cerebrovascular accidents, and, of course, dysphagia. The most marked change has been the increase in numbers of patients treated in nursing homes with a diagnosis of dysphagia. Currently, dysphagia accounts for the vast majority of nursing home caseload.

PATIENT/CLIENT PROFILE AND DISORDERS

According to ASHA, the average patient age is 77 years in a skilled-nursing facility and the average stay is 23 days, the average patient age is 67 years in a rehabilitation facility and the average stay is 20 days, and the average patient age is 74 years in home care and the average stay is 34 days. (ASHA, 2004a, 2004h, 2004i).

- The most common medical diagnoses among long-term-care patients seen by speech-language pathologist are
  - cardiovascular disease (40%),
  - respiratory disease (8%),
  - central nervous system (CNS) disorders (7%), and
  - transient ischemic attack (TIA; 5%).
- The most common medical diagnoses observed in the inpatient rehabilitation setting are
  - cerebrovascular disease (53%),
  - head injury (11%), and
  - hemorrhage/injury (6%).
- The most common medical diagnoses found in home health care are
  - cerebrovascular accidents (CVA; 58%),
  - central nervous system disease (CNS; 7%),
  - arterial occlusion or transient ischemic attack (TIA; 6%), and
  - respiratory distress (4%; ASHA, 2004a, 2004h, 2004i).

FINANCIAL RESOURCES

As we'll discuss in detail later, reimbursement (third-party payment) for speech-language pathology services in all three health-care settings overwhelmingly come from the Medicare system, which includes both Part A and Part B reimbursement. This means the therapist must have a strong understanding of the Medicare model. Most other payment systems (i.e., managed care, Medicaid), follow the Medicare model. Services require the following to submit for reimbursement:

- A physician's order.
- Signed treatment plan.
- The development of functional goals.

All reimbursement mechanisms are forms of cost containment, derived from a federal effort to reduce health-care costs. The speech-language pathologist with expertise has a strong understanding of the cost-containment mechanisms in the health-care setting.

COLLABORATION WITH COLLEAGUES VERSUS CROSS-TRAINING OF PROFESSIONALS

The expert speech-language pathologist must also know how to collaborate with other disciplines. This includes working effectively with an interdisciplinary team and finding numerous opportunities to interact with physical, occupational, and recreational therapists; physicians; nurses; social workers; dietitians; and others. The relationships established determine effectiveness in the work setting (ASHA, 2004a).

Most speech-language pathologists working in skilled-nursing facilities and home-care practice are contract employees—67% and 45%, respectively (ASHA, 2002a). Generally speaking, speech-language pathologists working in long-term-care facilities receive many requests for training other disciplines to provide their services for dysphagia rehabilitation. Typically, these requests reflect the scarcity of speech-language pathologists in these facilities. ASHA, however, has been quite clear in stating a policy against cross-training of other disciplines in dysphasia management (ASHA, 2004f).

Speech-language pathologists working in long-term care also typically work by themselves or with only one other speech-language pathologist. As a result, consultation with speech-language pathologists in other long-term-care environments becomes paramount to advanced speech language pathology/dysphagia treatment. Mentoring programs have gone a long way in eliminating feelings of isolation in the long-term-care arena. Some studies indicate that more than 72% of speech-language pathologist positions are unfilled. Frequently cited reasons for shortages were lack of qualified clinicians, low compensation, and undesirable work settings. Skilled-nursing facilities appear to have the greatest difficulties hiring qualified speech-language pathologists (ASHA, 2002a).

Speech-language pathologists in skilled-nursing facilities also tend to have the least professional supervision in the discipline. Speech-language pathologists working in home care also tend not to supervise many student speech-language pathologists in their health setting. Certainly, mentoring activities for novice clinicians in these settings could go a long way in stimulating recruitment efforts (ASHA, 2002a, b).

REGULATORY AND INSTITUTIONAL INFLUENCES

Three dramatic forces affect professional practitioners in these three settings. Like all health-care personnel, reimbursement (payment for services), policy-regulating agencies, and patient factors apply pressures within the skilled-nursing facility. The impact of reimbursement on treatment influences planning and effective treatment strategies. Shifts in health care relate to changes in reimbursement, regulatory demands, and factors within the patient population. Additional influences on reimbursement include the following:

- Balanced Budget Act of 1997.
- Private health insurance and managed health care.
- Lack of mandate by insurance carriers for speech, language, hearing, and swallowing disorders (Johnson, 2004).

Reimbursement Factors

Health-care cost-containment measures initially appeared in the 1980s with the advent of **diagnosis related groupings (DRGs)** in the hospital setting. Once cost-containment proved effective in that health-care setting, it was only a matter of time before other cost-containment mechanisms were applied. The Balanced Budget Act of 1997 introduced another form of cost-containment called the **prospective payment system** for a variety of health-care settings. While the prospective payment system differed between skilled-nursing facilities, inpatient or outpatient rehabilitation facilities, and home-care settings, the effect was to introduce cost-containment at different levels of the health-care continuum. Service delivery of treatment changed out of necessity. The frequency, intensity, and nature of speech pathology services changed under the prospective payment system in all three health-care settings. Most treatments are now offered only once a day rather than twice daily. Treatment duration shortened to make way for shared minutes with physical and occupational therapies.

The prospective payment system affects most levels of health care, regardless of treatment setting. In fact, by 2002, 95% of speech-language pathologists working in skilled-nursing facilities and 72% of those working in rehabilitation facilities indicated that they receive reimbursement under a form of payment influenced by the prospective payment system (ASHA, 2002a). The prospective payment system also influences how clinicians practice. For example, the prospective payment system is a per diem Part A payment mechanism, which can make use of additional instrumental assessments, such as modified barium swallow studies, difficult to justify. One study indicated that more than 50% of speech-language pathologists in the skilled-nursing facility experienced administrative pressure to limit use of instrumental swallowing studies for Medicare Part A patients due to the nature of the per diem reimbursement under the prospective payment system (ASHA, 2002a, b).

Currently, health care across all settings is experiencing dramatic change. Payment for service has changed from fee for service to **capitated** (maximum payment allowed for service) fees and other discounted arrangements, which are paid to the service providers.

Compounding the initiation of the prospective payment system was the capitation placed on Medicare Part B patients. Speech-language pathology services were also asked to share the capitated funds with physical therapy. As the amount of monies allocated typically amounted to approximately one month of treatment, the patient faced the dilemma of receiving within one year either therapy for physical mobility, communication, or swallowing under the Medicare Part B system. Patients who developed multiple problems within the year were in increased jeopardy. Skilled-nursing facilities were also at risk as they were legally bound to care for patients with multiple incidents during the year without adequate funding for their rehabilitation. Medicare Part B reimbursements remain an issue as of this writing. The federal government has yet to introduce an equitable plan for dealing with patients who exhibit complex, multiple disabilities or patients with multiple etiologies in the same calendar year. It is of critical importance for the expert to remain current on all aspects of reimbursement.

The speech-language pathologist in any of these health-care settings also faces an increasing number of patients with managed-care insurance programs. Managed care typically limits treatment access and duration as a form of cost-containment. Therapists, as a result, may have trouble acquiring treatment orders for some managed-care patients. The patient may be allotted fewer treatment sessions than needed to successfully complete the therapeutic regime.

Regulatory Factors

Public and private health-care institutions and agencies are typically governed by overseers who approve policies and procedures (ASHA, 2004b). Skilled-nursing facilities, rehabilitation facilities and home care are owned by private individuals or corporations. Most are owned by for-profit corporations, although some are not-for-profit businesses. Facilities approved for Medicare and Medicaid generally have governing bodies that approve institution policies and procedures and hire an administrator. These facilities are part of a highly regulated industry. Skilled-nursing and rehabilitation facilities are regulated by agencies such as those listed in Table 12.1.

Most states also provide a "report card" on each skilled-nursing facility that is available to the public. These methods of regulation are designed for the protection of the public. In addition, many of these health-care settings seek accreditation by the Community Health Accreditation Program, Incorporated (CHAP).

Speech-language pathologists are also regulated by their national professional organization. ASHA publishes documents to assist speech-language pathologists in regulating the practice. The most significant documents are the ASHA *Code of Ethics* and *Scope of Practice* (http://www.asha.org). Prudent speech-language pathologists carefully learn and adhere to the guidelines in these documents.

Federal and state governments have also continued to pass legislation that influences how health-care providers (including speech-language pathologists) respond to patients in a rehabilitation setting. The best example would be the federal legislation

TABLE 12.1 **Regulatory Bodies that Oversee Skilled-Nursing, Rehabilitation, and Home-Care Facilities**

Skilled-Nursing Facilities
Agency for Health Care Administration (AHCA)
Centers for Medicare and Medicaid Services (CMS)
Adult Protection Services
Children and Family Services
The Rehabilitation Accreditation Commission (CARF)
Joint Commission on Accreditation of Healthcare Organizations (JCAHO)
State Regulatory Agencies

Rehabilitation Facilities and Home-Care Agencies
Joint Commission on Health Care Organization (JACHO)
Centers for Medicare and Medicaid Services (CMS)
The Rehabilitation Accreditation Commission (CARF)
American Speech-Language-Hearing Association (ASHA)
Occupational Safety and Health Administration (OSHA)
State Regulatory Agencies
Community Health Accreditation Program, Inc. (CHAP): accrediting body for community health
   organizations including home health, hospice, and community rehabilitation centers.

passed to protect patient privacy and access to patient records, the Health Information Portability and Accountability Act (HIPAA). The speech-language pathologist with expertise maintains knowledge of ongoing federal and state regulatory legislation to ensure compliance with current legislation. Factors that influence legislation include federal, state, and local licensing bodies; health-care facility accreditation, credentialing entities; and institutional policies and procedures. Clinical competency, adequacy of documentation, quality of care, and measures of consumer satisfaction may relate to evaluation of ongoing competency development (ASHA, 2004b). See Table 12.2 for a sample check list for the development of clinical competencies in nursing homes, rehabilitation facilities, and home health-care agencies.

Patient Factors

In addition to the regulatory and reimbursement issues described previously, the speech-language pathologist is also influenced by patient factors. Patients seen in all three health-care settings are increasing in age because of life expectancy advances. The elderly population is also becoming more culturally diverse and more medically complex. The increased complexity can be explained in part by earlier discharges from acute-care facilities. In addition, advanced technology has significantly influenced mortality rates over the past decade, although patients tend to have a multiplicity of diagnoses and functional declines. The patients are also much more aware of their *patient rights* and advocate for superior health care by assuming a more active role in health-care decisions (ASHA, 2004b).

Reimbursement, regulatory, and patient factors are requiring speech-language pathologists to modify staffing patterns, service delivery, and patient management. Changes in staffing patterns include the following:

- Per-visit treatment time has decreased, which can change overall treatment duration as well as increase individual clinician's patient caseload.
- Productivity expectations are raised by increasing demands for "billable" treatment opportunities.
- Employers may want to hire more part-time staff to reduce costs and employee benefits. Therapists may be expected to work in several facilities. Speech-language pathologists may be asked to assume more administrative, case management, and data entry responsibilities (ASHA, 2004b).

TABLE 12.2 Sample Competency Checklist-Validation

Competency reassessment, an ongoing unit-collaborative assessment of competency, is site specific, department specific, and job specific. Competency is based on three domains.

- *Critical Thinking*: Focuses clinical simulations that verify clinical judgment.
- *Technical Skills*: Collaboratively identifying high-risk/high-frequency and high-risk/low-frequency procedures.
- *Interpersonal Skills*: Focuses on written or verbal communication and how to resolve conflict.

Competencies are DUE _____

Name _____ Job Title _____ Date _____

Mandatories	Date	Renewal Date	Validator	Comments
Education				
CPR				
License Renewal				
CCC Renewal				

Ongoing Competencies *These are hospital/unit-related initiatives based on the track and trending data previously collected and identified by the Performance Improvement Department as necessary.*

Date	How Met	Age-Specific Knowledge/ Competence & Skills	Infant	Child	Adult	Geriatric
		Normal vs. pathological processes in growth, development, and aging.				
		Professional skills in gathering objective age-specific data used to evaluate, assess, & treat.				
		Displays procedures for safety & infection control				
		Operates equipment				
		Interprets monitoring equipment & data collection in all treatment areas related to age.				
		Communicates effective age-based information to family/caregiver regarding (a) speech-language & dysphagia diagnosis/treatment (b) home exercise or functional maintenance program (c) specific precautions related to feeding/swallowing (d) involves patient and caregiver in PLAN OF CARE.				
		Can identify abuse and neglect				
		Knowledge of proper referral				
		Knowledge of funding sources: HMO, Medicare, Medicaid, & clinical relevance to patient				
		Demonstrates correct procedure for applying or removing chest & wrist constraints				

Summary

The employee needs to complete the following Action Plan

- Provide proof of attendance at educational program(s)
- Read policies on _____ and complete post-test.
- Submit written summary of article(s) on _____
- Complete skill demonstration on _____
- Submit written case study exemplar on _____

Comments:

The employee will be reassessed on the competencies on _____ (date)

Employee meets _____ Does not meet _____ the above competency

If corrective action is needed, a corrective/remediation action plan will be implemented.

_____   _____

Manager Signature   **Date**

_____   _____

Employee Signature   **Date**

Service delivery may be affected in the following ways:

- Limits are applied to twice-daily treatments (BID) and individual sessions.
- Under prospective payment system (PPS) guidelines, service delivery is regulated regarding treatment length, frequency, and duration (ASHA, 2004b).

Patient management may be affected in the following ways:

- Speech-language pathologists must document skilled, medically necessary services in clear and functional terms. Documentation guidelines are discussed later in this chapter.
- Emphasis on caregiver and/or family education is increasing.
- Emphasis is increasing on remediation to reach *functional status* of patients, requiring measurement and demonstrating outcomes (ASHA, 2004b).
- Dysphagia management presents a particular challenge under PPS because of staff involvement, facility responsibility for instrumental examinations, and treatment modalities (thickened liquids, altered diets), as well as the cost of dysphagia management by a speech-language pathologist.

Speech-language pathologists must remain open to changing and expanding roles. Focus is increasing regarding counseling and training for families, proficiency in data collection for outcome measures, and increased reliance of technology. Other changes may include more active involvement as case managers, rehabilitation directors, or marketing experts (ASHA, 2004b).

INDICATORS OF EXPERTISE IN THE THREE WORK SETTINGS

The speech-language pathologist requires only a state license in most states. In most instances, speech-language pathologists must also accrue continuing education credit to maintain their state license. In states with professional licensure, ASHA Certificate of Clinical Competence (CCC) status may be voluntary. Also voluntary is any ASHA specialty recognition board certification, such as board certification in dysphagia. While participation in national and board certification may be voluntary, it serves to distinguish individuals with expertise from those with general professional preparation. ASHA documents assist speech-language pathologists in determining and refining roles and competencies. The technical report, *Provision of Audiology and Speech-Language Pathology Services to Older Persons in Nursing Homes* reviews therapist roles in long-term-care settings (ASHA, 1988). ASHA documents that assist speech-language pathologists in determining their competencies include the following:

- *Roles of Speech-Language Pathologists in Swallowing and Feeding Disorders* (ASHA, 2002b)
- *Knowledge and Skills Needed by Speech-Language Pathologists Providing Services to Individuals with Cognitive-Communication Disorders* (ASHA, 2005)
- *Knowledge and Skills in Business Practices Needed by Speech-Language Pathologists in Health Care Settings* (ASHA, 2003)

Most of these documents may be found on the American Speech-Language Hearing Association website (http://www.asha.org).

Many health-care facilities, as well as contract companies serving long-term-care, rehabilitation, and home-care facilities have a competency checklist for nursing and rehabilitation professionals working there. The competency checklist is usually completed at hiring and updated with the annual review. The competency checklist assesses understanding of policy and procedures as well as regulatory compliance. The checklist also assesses basic knowledge and skills in the areas of dysphagia management, assessments and treatment of disorders such as receptive and expressive language and cognitive disorders, and augmentative communication devices. The competency checklists are designed to establish *basic* competency to perform duties and rarely identify exceptional or advanced competency. See Table 12.2 for a sample checklist of competencies.

A few health-care providers use the title senior speech-language pathologist or speech-language pathologist Level II. Most do not recognize advanced competency via title, although some offer enhanced compensation packages. Some long-term-care companies employ clinical consultants to work with physical, occupational, and speech-language pathologists to improve clinical skills and documentation/coding abilities. The clinical consultant may be a member of any of the disciplines and, as a result, may not completely understand the clinical needs of a therapist from a different discipline. For this reason, some health-care providers have developed a speech-mentoring program to address the specific needs of speech-language pathologists working in long-term care. These mentoring programs may provide free regional ASHA-approved continuing education credit workshops. The workshops range from topics such as dysphagia management, neurogenic disorders, aural rehabilitation, documentation and coding, and functional goal-writing skills. This helps to satisfy the need for life-long learning, as well as the need to obtain continuing education credits to maintain a state license.

In addition, new employees may receive one-on-one professional mentoring. Novice speech-language pathologists are assigned a mentor who has received advanced training through a *train the trainer* program. The mentor works with each new speech-language pathologist to ensure success in therapy. Each mentoring experience is different; the mentored therapist creates a list of topics or procedures to learn. This list becomes a contract between the mentor and the novice speech-language pathologist. The mentor does not report to the immediate supervisor of the novice, allowing the novice to feel more comfortable honestly expressing weaknesses in various clinical areas. The novice clinician also has a lifeline to the mentor for ongoing clinical assistance for as long as needed. The program maintains a hotline for therapists to call with clinical questions, forwarding questions to specialists in the particular field of care. Thus, the mentoring program helps the novice establish a strong foundation at the beginning of employment, provides ongoing education, and, most important, the mentoring program offers ongoing clinical support for speech-language pathologists in the field.

Novice speech-language pathologists may not be beginning their clinical fellowship. Many professionals with years of experience in other clinical settings, such as the school system or private practice may need retooling to change employment settings. The ability to change work setting or specialization is a positive outcome within this profession. Ample opportunities for continuing education and retooling are available.

The pursuit of expertise can also occur outside of the workplace through continuing education opportunities. Many areas in the country have local study groups where professionals gather to master or refine a particular subject. Monthly meetings may rotate among various facilities to enhance participation in a wide range of topical discussions and lectures. State associations also offer cost-effective continuing education credit. Certainly, continuing education is also available at many associations' national meetings and conventions. In addition, speech-language pathologists find continuing education at local universities, including advanced certificates to increase knowledge beyond the master's degree. These specialty programs may increase the likelihood that participants will achieve ASHA board specialty recognition.

TREATMENT EFFICACY AND EXPERTISE

Nursing homes, rehabilitation facilities, community-based service providers, and home-health agencies, like other health-care settings, have tried to apply treatment modalities derived from evidence-based practice. The long-term-care community has traditionally not taken the lead in and the establishment of evidence based practice. Most investigations have taken place at the university level to accommodate the need for randomized controlled clinical trials. This type of clinical trial is typically not available in the long-term-care, rehabilitation, and home-care environments. Speech-language pathologists working in these environments look to university personnel to define evidence-based practice in communication disorders. Their response to the research is generally positive and produces changes in the treatment modalities used in their environments (ASHA, 2004c).

Treatment-efficacy data collection is becoming more common. (See Chapter 7 for additional information on treatment efficacy and evidenced-based practice.) Health-care facilities recognize that collecting treatment efficacy data can positively influence payment/funding sources and, as a result, reimbursement for their services. This outcome data can become an influential instrument for insurance company negotiation and consumer advocacy. The result can be increased third-party coverage for speech and dysphagia services, improved quality care for patients, enhanced patient success, and as a useful tool for staffing within the facility (ASHA, 2004g).

ASHA established the National Outcomes Measurement System (NOMS) in 1997 to collect outcomes data from a variety of health-care settings. NOMS was developed to demonstrate the value of clinical services provided for adults and children with communication and swallowing disorders. NOMS quantification requires **functional communication measures (FCM)**. FCMs are based on a seven-point rating scale specific to types of disorders and designed to describe the change in an individual's functional communication ability (ASHA, 2004g).

Clinicians do not administer any special assessments or withhold treatment for any patients but collect data as treatment begins and when treatment ends and the patient is discharged. The information obtained includes diagnoses, demographics, functional status, clinical setting, amount, frequency and intensity of services, and discharge disposition (ASHA, 2004g). ASHA has published treatment efficacy summaries based on the outcome data. The treatment efficacy summary for swallowing disorders, for example, states that postural techniques eliminated thin liquid aspiration in approximately 80% of the patients. Pharyngeal muscle strengthening exercises also resulted in increased swallowing (ASHA, 2004i).

NOMS, for speech-language pathologists working in skilled-nursing facilities, demonstrated that patients at FCM Level 3 for swallowing disorder (maintaining less than 50% of nutrition and hydration by mouth) needed increased treatment time to achieve better functional outcomes. Patient progress to a Level 5 (all nutrition and hydration with minimal diet restrictions such as soft foods or nectar thick liquids) required almost twice the amount of treatment needed to reach Level 4 (ASHA, 2004d, 2004g).

COMMONALITIES IN ALL HEALTH-CARE SETTINGS

Certain knowledge and skills are essential across *all* health-care settings. Speech-language pathologists must master them to achieve expertise in their field. These commonalities include

1. Expert knowledge of anatomy and physiology
2. Documentation and coding
3. Basic business knowledge and practices

Expert Knowledge and Skills

Each speech-language pathologist with expertise has a strong grounding in anatomy and physiology. Whether the expertise is in dysphagia, aphasia, voice, or other disorders, all diagnostic and treatment skills are based not only on knowledge of basic anatomy but more importantly on a strong understanding of the physiology of the disorder. Without this knowledge base, the speech-language pathologist in any health-care setting could not design treatment modalities with competence. Unfortunately, many practitioners in all health-care settings have only a cursory knowledge of anatomy and physiology. For this reason, mentoring programs often emphasize a review of anatomy and physiology of the speech and swallowing mechanism. One-on-one mentoring may also emphasize increased skill in this area. These structures and processes are considered requirements to understanding the necessary support mechanisms for advanced therapeutic strategies.

Documentation and Coding

Another skill common to all health-care settings is the ability to properly document and code therapy services, which must be mastered if the speech-language pathologist is to be considered an expert. Speech-language pathologists who work with adults with communication and swallowing problems must understand Medicare regulations and provide documentation that supports needs for and benefit of clinical services (Swigert, 2002). Fiscal intermediaries frequently report the need to improve and upgrade documentation and coding abilities. Personnel who review charts for insurance companies have stated that documentation quality is frequently so poor that they cannot recommend funding or overturning a denial even though they believe it appropriate (Johnson, 2003). Proper documentation and accurate coding for services can significantly increase the potential for timely payment and decrease the probability of a denial. Therefore, speech-language pathologists and audiologists need to achieve mastery of proper documentation and coding (Johnson, 2004).

Documentation provides an important running record of clinical care. This record provides a means of communication for health-care professionals, billing documentation, proof of quality improvement and compliance, research data collection, and legal evidence. Medicare has defined key principles to guide accurate documentation; these are briefly defined in Table 12.3.

Understanding what and how to document is critical, as it forms the basis for payment of services. Unfortunately for the profession, a Department of Health and Human Services report concluded that fourteen percent of skilled-nursing facility rehabilitation services were unnecessary based on poor documentation presented (Swigert, 2002). The expert speech-language pathologist knows the patient's insurance company description of medical necessity when requesting authorization for services. The documentation must clearly indicate *why* the therapeutic intervention is appropriate for this patient's medical condition (Kummer, Johnson, & Zeit, in press).

The process of documentation can be expensive and time-consuming. The speech-language pathologist with expertise must determine how to stay abreast of new Medicare and local fiscal intermediary changes in policy to ensure compliance with standards and, at the same time, complete documentation in a cost-effective manner. This is certainly true when, in most health-care settings, the time and effort spent in documentation is not

TABLE 12.3   Key Principles as Defined by Medicare for Accurate Documentation

Key Principles	Defined
Medical Necessity	Critical for patient survival
Change of Condition	Documentation of improvement or decline in patient's condition.
Previous Level of Function (PLF)	Documentation of patient's premorbid function, abilities, and previous interventions.
Reasonable and Necessary	Duration and frequency of therapeutic services are appropriate.
Specific	Treatment goals & methods are based on FCM.
Effective	Expectation that treatment will improve patient's condition.
Skilled	Treatment strategies are complex and require advanced/expert skills.
Functional and Measurable Goals	Activities must be functional to the patient's improved outcomes and be quantifiable over time.

directly billable. For this reason many experts are turning to technology. More health-care settings are using computerized documentation to create more streamlined and efficient documentation procedures (Kummer, 2004).

The experienced speech-language pathologist also understands the need to remain current in proper coding. The Centers for Medicare and Medicaid (CMS) and the American Medical Association (AMA) review codes on a consistent basis. CMS publishes the quarterly *Correct Coding Initiative* (*CCI*). This federal document is essential reading to maintain compliance with coding regulation. The fiscal intermediaries interpret CMS direction and publish local medical review policies listing allowable codes for specific disorders. It is important to note, however, that most local medical review policies lists of codes are not all-inclusive. A main function of the ASHA Health Care Economics Committee is to advocate for proper codes for speech, language, hearing, and swallowing disorders. The speech-language pathologist with expertise will check on developments in federal- and local-level coding at least quarterly.

The expert also works with other therapists to ensure proper coding procedures and instructs other therapists that it is their responsibility to *code to the level of the therapeutic procedures* utilized in each session. He or she also instructs others that it is also the therapist's responsibility to *document to accurately reflect therapeutic procedures used within the session*. Documentation requires constant searching for better ways to meet the needs of the customers, demonstrate the value of our services, and maintain timely performance (Kummer, Johnson, & Zeit, in press).

KNOWLEDGE OF BUSINESS AND PRACTICE

The other common trait found among speech-language pathologists who seek excellence and expertise in their profession is their understanding of business practices. The practice of speech language pathology is a business. The advanced professional (whether solo or in a large rehabilitation department) cannot approach practice-related decisions without considering health-care financial management concepts. In a successful business, our income must balance our expenses. Furthermore, we need to reinvest in our business to remain solvent and provide the necessary services to our clients (Kummer, 2004). Several years ago, ASHA recognized that speech-language pathology needed to become more familiar with business practices. As a result, Alex Johnson, Ph.D., vice president for professional practices in speech language pathology assembled a committee on business practice. The committee developed two knowledge and skills documents, *Knowledge and Skills in Business Practices Needed by Speech-Language Pathologists in Health Care Settings* (ASHA, 2003) and *Knowledge and Skills in Business Practices for Speech-Language Pathologists Who Are Managers and Leaders in Healthcare Organizations* (ASHA, 2004e). These documents informed speech-language pathologists about business concepts but gave them no resource for learning those concepts. An ASHA-sponsored book, *Business Matters: A Guide for Speech-Language Pathologists* (Golper & Brown, 2004) discusses many key elements of management related to speech-language pathology. Key elements of business practices are discussed next.

Leadership

Leadership encompasses understanding organizational processes and personal and organizational goals. Factors such as leadership roles, motivation, strategic planning, organizational missions, and company values must be addressed to gain expertise in this area.

Service Delivery

Today's health-care environment requires delivery of the highest quality clinical services in a cost-effective manner (Golper & Brown, 2004). To understand service delivery, the speech-language pathologist seeking to gain expertise must understand concepts such as operating margins, productivity targets, reimbursements (including Medicare, Medicaid, insurance, managed care, and private pay), documentation and coding (including CPT, ICD codes), and ethical practice, as well as resource utilization.

Financial Management

Businesses must be financially responsible in their operation. Organizations operate within a budget and have fiscal responsibilities (Golper & Brown, 2004). The speech-language pathologist desiring expertise in financial management needs to be well-versed in budgets, revenue streams, profit motives, cost analysis, types of corporations available for businesses as well as general accounting principles.

Standards and Compliance

Experts have legal and ethical obligations to comply with professional and regulatory standards. Speech-language pathologists desiring expertise in this area would need to understand policies and procedures; corporate compliance; credentialing and accreditations; risk management; privacy issues; confidentiality issues and conflicts of interest.

Quality and Performance Improvements

Experts must go beyond minimal standards and develop knowledge beyond entry-level requirements. The speech-language pathologist with expertise understands how to analyze quality within the work setting. **Quality** refers to achieving the highest possible clinical outcomes for the patients. Quality is reflected in employee satisfaction, customer satisfaction, retention of both employees and customers, and strong financial performance. We associate the following features with quality:

- Consistency and dependability.
- Responsiveness to employees and consumers.
- Competence.
- Respectful and considerate treatment.
- Safety.
- Accessibility.
- Ethical treatments.
- Excellent communication.

Technology

Professionals seeking expertise apply technology appropriately in the work setting. They discover what technology is available and have a keen sense how it can be applied. Technology and advanced knowledge of it improve our work quality, accuracy, cost-effectiveness, efficiency, and speed.

Personnel Management

Successful business leaders recognize that valued and satisfied employees are productive and less likely to leave the organization. Leaders understand that it is less costly to retain experienced and skilled personnel than to train novices repeatedly (Golper & Brown, 2004). An expert understands employee job descriptions and how to administer a work-flow analysis. The organization's staffing plan should be realistic and include hiring opportunities for contingency situations. A recruitment process should be in place and functioning. In addition, new-employee orientation should be comprehensive and represent employer expectations clearly and realistically. Competencies must be defined and established before clinical treatment, and continuing education and training should focus on needed areas of employee development.

Marketing

Marketing strategies can improve performance, enhance competition, and increase customer satisfaction. The expert in marketing knows the elements of market research such as market analysis, competition analysis, and consumer analysis. A speech-language pathology practice can develop its marketing "mix" by looking at its unique combination of price, product, place, and promotion. From that, a strong and well-thought-out marketing plan can be developed.

Advocacy

Experts have learned that they must encourage others to recognize how their professional services improve patient outcome. They must demonstrate *how* services improve quality of life and reduce the impact of the disorder. The professional seeking expertise in this area needs to understand how legislative and regulatory processes work and the value of coalition networks as well as the different types of advocacy. Probably the most important aspect of advocacy is to understand how to advocate for a cause.

All of the concepts presented are discussed in detail in the book, *Business Matters: A Guide for Speech-Language Pathologists* (Golper & Brown, 2004). Each chapter also provides business principles, references, resources, and real-life examples. It is designed to help speech-language pathologists gain expertise to help ensure the survival of their practice as well as the survival of our profession.

 ## SUMMARY

Speech-language pathologists practicing in any health-care environment must recognize the need for clinical expertise. The pursuit of expertise is a lifelong path that begins with willingness to commit oneself to the journey. Persistence and pursuit of expertise yield benefits for the speech-language pathologist and patients, as well as for long-term-care, rehabilitation, and community-based service providers. The professional soon learns that the journey itself can be just as rewarding as finally reaching the goal of expertise.

 ## THOUGHTS FOR EXPLORATION

1. What skills are unique to practice in long-term-care settings?
2. What impact can funding have on a patient's rate of progress?
3. What communication disorders can the speech-language pathologist anticipate treating in any of the long-term-care facilities whether with in-patient or out-patient clients?

REFERENCES

American Speech-Language-Hearing Association. (1988, March). *Provision of audiology and speech-language pathology services to older persons in nursing homes* (pp. 772–774). Rockville, MD: Author.

American Speech-Language-Hearing Association. (2002a). *Speech-language pathology health care survey.* Rockville, MD: Author.

American Speech-Language-Hearing Association. (2002b, April 16). Roles of speech-language pathologists in swallowing and feeding disorders: Position statement. *ASHA Leader, 7* (Suppl. 22), 73.

American Speech-Language-Hearing Association. (2003). *Knowledge and skills in business practice needed by speech-language pathologists in health care settings. ASHA Supplement, 23,* 87–92.

American Speech-Language-Hearing Association. (2004a). *Getting started in long-term care.* Available at http://www.asha.org/members/slp/healthcare/start_long.htm

American Speech-Language-Hearing Association. (2004b). *Health care issues brief-long term care.* Available at http://www.asha.org/members/slp/healthcare/long_term.htm

American Speech-Language-Hearing Association. (2004c). *Evidence-based practice in communication disorders: an introduction* (Tech. Rep.). Available at http://www.asha.org/members/deskref-journals/deskref/default

American Speech-Language-Hearing Association. (2004d). *SLP treatment outcomes in skilled nursing.* Adult NOMS Fact Sheet. Rockville, MD: Author.

American Speech-Language-Hearing Association. (2004e). *Knowledge and skills in business practices for speech-language pathologists who are managers and leaders in health care organizations. ASHA Supplement,* 24.

American Speech-Language-Hearing Association. (2004f). Speech-language pathologists training and supervising other professionals in the delivery of services to individuals with swallowing and feeding disorders. Position Statement. *ASHA Supplement,* 24.

American Speech-Language-Hearing Association. (2004g). *About NOMS.* Available at http://www.asha.org/members/research/NOMS/about_noms.htm

American Speech-Language-Hearing Association. (2004h). *Getting started in acute inpatient rehabilitation.* Available at http://www.asha.org/members.slp/healthcare/start_acute_in.htm

American Speech-Language-Hearing Association. (2004i). *Treatment efficacy summary: Swallowing disorders (dysphagia) in adults.* Rockville MD: Author.

American Speech-Language-Hearing Association. (2005). *Knowledge and skills needed by speech-language pathologists providing services to individuals with cognitive-communication disorders. ASHA Supplement,* 25.

Golper, L. A., & Brown, J. (Eds.). (2004). *Business matters: A guide for speech-language pathologists.* Rockville, MD: American Speech-Language-Hearing Association.

Johnson, P. R. (2003). Entry level business practice knowledge and skills document. *ASHA Perspectives on Administration and Supervision, 13*(1), 10–11.

Johnson, P. R. (2004). Documentation and coding for improved reimbursement. *ASHA Perspectives on Administration and Supervision, 14*(2), 7–9.

Kummer, A. W. (2004). Speech-language pathology: It's our business. *ASHA Perspectives on Administration and Supervision, 14*(3), 9–11.

Kummer, A. W., Johnson, P. R., & Zeit, K. (2006). Clinical documentation in medical speech-language pathology. In A. Johnson (Ed.), *Medical speech-language pathology.* Strow, OH: Interactive Therapeutics.

Swigert, N. (2002, February 5). Documenting what you do is as important as doing it. *ASHA Leader, 7*(2), 14–17.

CHAPTER 13

Speech-Language Pathology in Medical Settings

Alex Johnson

Acute Care   Care typically provided by professionals in hospital and outpatient facilities; generally the most immediate care. Upon completion of acute care management, the patient is either dismissed or transferred into long-term care.

INTRODUCTION

Speech-language pathologists work in many types of medical settings, including acute care and rehabilitation hospitals, nursing and extended-care facilities, and outpatient clinics associated with these institutions. The scope of work in these settings varies even more than the settings themselves. Speech-language pathologists in medical settings see children and adults, provide services to patients with nearly every type of communication or swallowing disorder, and use special technologies unique to the medical setting.

VALUE OF THE SERVICES PROVIDED

Before we enter a technical discussion of medical speech-language pathology practice, it may be helpful to discuss the value of the services provided in this rich context. Speech-language pathologists in hospitals and other medical settings have an exceptional privilege, the opportunity to bring focus to speech, language, and swallowing needs of patients who have widely varying medical complaints. In this setting, speech-language pathologists evaluate individual patients; consult for physicians in charge of patient primary medical care, deliver treatment services to help reduce the medical condition's effects and provide rehabilitation, and, as the patient's condition advances, to bring attention to long-term rehabilitation needs and supports.

ROLES AND RESPONSIBILITIES

Activities in medical speech-language pathology practices vary by setting (acute care versus outpatient care), specialty focus (geriatric medicine versus pediatric medicine), and the type of practice model employed (direct service versus consultative service). Each of these variables, and many others, dictate the scope of clinical activities employed, as well as the type of clinical interactions with other providers. Speech-language pathologists entering medical settings might prefer the fast-paced and diverse practice in the typical large acute-care environment to the steadier-paced and "scheduled" environment of the rehabilitation hospital or outpatient center.

Clinicians in *all* medical practice styles and settings conduct their professional activities to the highest standards of professional practice, become familiar with institutional operating procedures and ethical guidelines, and provide efficient and safe care for patients. Uninformed or unskilled practitioners in health settings place patients at significant health risk, increasing the risk of **medical errors,** and reflect poorly on the profession. Thus, speech-language pathologists in the medical setting have an obligation to keep current in their clinical skills and knowledge and to seek adequate supervision and training to ensure that their clinical skills are the best that they can be.

The nature of medical speech-language pathology services requires unique abilities in communication and interpersonal relationships, professional skills and knowledge, awareness of specific ethical and competency standards, as well as a relatively thorough understanding of disease conditions and their effect on communication and swallowing. In this chapter, we review some of these topics and issues.

A complete review of medical speech-language pathology is beyond the scope of this chapter. Extensive reviews of medical setting-specific information can be found in texts by Golper (1998), Johnson and Jacobson (1998), and Miller and Groher (1990). Each of these resources, while taking a different focus, emphasizes key features of medical speech-language pathology practice including content (clinical) information, interprofessional relationships, and highly specific skills and knowledge.

CHANGING WORLD OF MEDICAL SPEECH-LANGUAGE PATHOLOGY

Various influences inform and shape speech-language pathology practice in any given setting. Examples of these influences include culture, financial and regulatory issues, and technology.

As the culture changes, new demands and opportunities arise. Examples of cultural shifts that have influenced medical speech-language pathology practice include increased need for services by people from many linguistic and ethnic backgrounds, and increased energy directed at providing services for patients to the end of life. Because of the diversity of clinical speech-language practica opportunities in educational programs, few new graduates have extensive experience in health-care needs in cultures other than their own. Thus, most new clinicians need extensive supervision and guided observation in medical settings before initiating any level of independent practice. New graduates seeking employment in these settings should be assured that more-experienced practitioners will provide necessary instruction and guidance to develop essential competencies and to ensure patient safety.

Reimbursement

In addition to issues of culture, political-legal-financial aspects of care have changed dramatically in the past decade. The shift from a fee–for-service health care model to one increasingly based on capitation (maximum amount that can be charged to third-party payers) or other managed-care models has prompted much change in speech-language pathology practice. These changes included reduced length of stay in inpatient settings, reduced reimbursement rates for certain conditions, reductions in the amount of time (or number of visits) a patient can be seen for treatment and so forth. These "realities" have caused considerable concern among providers and patients; however, they have led clinicians to impressive attempts to improve care despite cutbacks in financial support through use of new therapy models, inclusion of assistants and families as therapy "extenders," improving priorities and goal setting activities, and demonstrating intervention outcomes. For an excellent review of information regarding the business aspects of medical speech-language pathology, refer to Golper and Brown (2004). Speech-language pathologists beginning practice in medical settings should make every effort to learn about reimbursement requirements, documentation practices, and coding of patient conditions and services. They must understand the financial ramifications of the services they provide. In health-care settings, speech-language pathology services (and all skilled services) are typically expensive, and every clinician should appreciate the implications for patients of each decision and clinical practice.

Advocacy

These practical issues in medical clinical practice call for every clinician to advocate for their patients. When the speech-language pathologist views services as essential for the patient's benefit and those services are denied for reasons of reimbursement or other arbitrary rationales, the speech-language pathologist must communicate patient needs and potential benefits of the service to decision makers. Frequently, reimbursement decision makers are physicians or nurses who may lack familiarity with speech-language pathology practice and its associated risks and benefits. Skilled clinicians with strong advocacy skills can often change the minds of decision makers through careful, respectful, and clear communication. Advocacy for patients by talented clinicians can ultimately determine whether or not a patient receives the treatment services necessary for a desirable outcome.

Technology

Practice technologies have also changed dramatically. In the past 20 years, the use of computer technology for all aspects of practice has increased dramatically. In many institutions, access to the patient's medical record demands basic computer literacy. Additionally, speech-language pathologists are frequently involved in clinical activities that demand a high standard of performance in either using technology or interpreting data from technical sources. A brief list of these activities with references can be found in Table 13.1. Rarely does one clinician have expertise in all of these skill areas. Each demands training and supervised experience typically acquired in postsecondary educational and continuing education experiences.

Many of the technologies listed in Table 13.1 can impose risk to patients when applied inappropriately. Clinicians should always put the needs of their patient first and provide only high-risk services for which they are qualified. For example, ASHA has provided guidelines for the use of fiber-optic endoscopic instrumentation in evaluating vocal function or swallowing (ASHA, 2004). These guidelines outline the elements of safe and effective use of endoscopy, and clinicians should comply with these

TABLE 13.1   Examples of the Technical Aspects of Speech-Language Pathology

Technology	Typical Use in SLP	Reference
Videofluoroscopy	Swallowing studies	Logemann (1998)
Videostroboscopy	Voice assessment	Karnell & Langmore (1998)
Fiber-Optic Endoscopy	Swallowing assessment	Karnell & Langmore (1998)
Electromyography	Voice, motor speech	Karnell (1989)
Ultrasound	Swallowing study	Chi Fishman & Sonies (2002)
Functional Imaging of Brain	Language and cognitive assessments	George, Vikingstad, & Cao (1998)
Cortical Stimulation	Language localization before or during surgery	Valachovic, Smith, Elisevich, Jacobson, & Fisk (1998)

guidelines when carrying out the procedure. When clinicians fail to follow professional standards of practice they may place themselves at risk if the patient suffers an adverse effect.

COMMUNICATION IN THE MEDICAL SETTING

The communication demands exerted on the speech-language pathologist in medical settings are complex. Clinicians must communicate regularly and well with other disciplines (e.g., physicians, nurses, pharmacists, technicians, etc.), families and patients, colleagues in the discipline, and administrators. In addition, they must be efficient and effective in oral communication, written notes, and electronic forms of communication.

While excellent oral and written communication skills are hallmarks of all good speech-language pathology practice, the medical setting offers unique communication demands and situations. These have been organized around two topics: effective consultation and difficult communication situations.

Effective Consultation

In many medical settings, especially acute-care facilities, the primary service may be consultation. In this model the clinician receives a patient on referral from a physician; evaluates, interviews, and observes the patient; provides recommendations for follow up; and provides interventions focused on immediate patient needs. This model has become increasingly common with short patient stays and reduced staffing patterns in many acute-care hospitals in the United States and Canada.

Lee, Pappius, and Goldman (1983) identified the three most common reasons that referring physicians request a consultation: advice regarding a diagnosis, advice regarding management, and assistance in completing a test or procedure. A timely response to a request for consultation is an essential component of good patient care. Speech-language pathologists have information useful in helping the physician clarify symptoms that may contribute to the diagnosis. Skilled description of language-processing characteristics, motor speech or voice symptoms, oral motor capabilities, or developmental characteristics can provide a window into the patient's problem not otherwise accessible to the physician or other referral source. Speech-language pathologists sometimes forget that not all physicians, nurses, and psychologists have extensive experience in speech, language, or swallowing diagnosis.

Typically, following a consultation, the speech-language pathologist generates a written consultation report. Such reports are brief, specific, and informative. Examples of written consultation reports for acute care can be found in Johnson, Valachovic, and George (1998).

Communicating in Difficult Situations

Many patients and their families are upset, anxious, fatigued, or distressed during the acute stage of recovery or the rehabilitative process. It does not take extensive imagination to quickly empathize with the needs of our patients. Although our awareness and sensitivity might be finely attuned to our patients' requirements, we need to develop specific skills to interact most effectively. The discussion of interpersonal characteristics in Chapter 5 offers suggestions for developing and using those specific skills. Failure to communicate well in these situations can compromise the relationship with patients, families, and referral sources. At worst, failed communication with patients can lead to serious legal or disciplinary consequences.

What are these "difficult" communication situations for the speech-language pathologist? First and foremost, the issue of dealing with those who are angry, emotionally upset, or otherwise confrontational is not a topic well covered in many graduate programs.

Many clinicians might have their first experience with this on the job. Novice clinicians should identify strong clinical role models and mentors and not be reticent to seek their advice in these situations. In many institutions, a clinical social worker, psychologist, or pastoral professional can provide sound guidance and also assist in dealing directly with difficult situations. With experience and focus, speech-language pathologists learn to deal with these situations with great skill.

A second difficult communication situation occurs when the speech-language pathologist must deliver bad news to the patient or family. These communications rarely focus on life and death, rather the situation more typically involves discussing a potential or impending loss of function (e.g., communication, swallowing), need for difficult or prolonged treatment, or making a life adjustment as the result of a serious communication or swallowing disturbance. Each of these situations requires great skill in listening as much as in talking. Again, spending time observing experienced professionals, using appropriate caution and sensitivity, and learning to avoid projection of your own sense of loss, hopelessness, or anxiety onto the patient are key elements of developing this important skill set.

It follows that communication skills are essential to good practice and especially critical in the consultative role of the clinical practitioner. These skills provide the professional "envelope" in which relationships are established and maintained. Successful communication involves deliberate and focused delivery of messages directed at enhancing understanding of the patient's problem and the treatment options available. Patient and referral source satisfaction increase significantly when clinicians effectively relay information, deliver both good and bad news, and share their rationale for various decisions.

Johnson and Jacobson (1998) provide a list of significant errors in medical speech-language pathology practice. Many of these errors relate to failures in oral and written communication. Some common/frequent examples include failure to:

- Communicate results of a high-risk or invasive procedure accurately or in a timely manner.
- Document detailed recommendations in the chart (especially diet changes or aspiration precautions).
- Respond to referrals or information requests in a timely manner, especially when this delay causes interruption of care.
- Communicate results of the speech-language or swallowing evaluation.
- Document significant changes in patient behavior.
- Make diagnostic statements or conclusions substantiated by observations or data.
- Follow up on recommendations previously documented.
- Document and explain important information to the family.
- Ensure confidentiality of patient information.

This list is not exhaustive, but it offers guidance regarding the significance and risk associated with communication in health-care settings.

PROFESSIONAL SKILLS AND KNOWLEDGE

The specific skills and knowledge needed for medical speech-language pathology can be divided into two categories: general and specialty. General information includes all of the basic competencies required for the ASHA Certificate of Clinical Competence (ASHA, 2004), additional setting-specific knowledge, and service delivery knowledge. Setting-specific knowledge includes the operating characteristics of the program in which you are working, requirements for infection control, and any special procedures or technologies in use. A second area of setting-specific information relates to knowledge associated with patient populations you are likely to encounter most frequently. For example, the knowledge requirements for conducting a basic speech and language assessment in the intensive-care unit of a large teaching hospital are considerably different from evaluating a patient recovering from a head injury in an outpatient setting. In both of these examples, the speech-language pathologist is obligated to do the following:

- Understand the basic mechanisms of the underlying disease process or injury.
- Appreciate the prognosis for the condition.
- Know the impact and significance of any medications or other procedures in use.
- Understand the mental and emotional status of the patient relative to the current condition.

Each of these areas of information is essential to patient management in that setting. The variability in types of patients seen in diverse medical settings requires the clinician to learn common medical diagnoses of patients seen in the particular setting and to learn about the likely treatments and **sequelae** (aftereffects) associated with the disease or injury.

In addition to these basic (universal) knowledge requirements for speech-language pathologists in medical settings, clinicians must develop necessary "specialized" skills for the populations they serve. In this case, "specialized" refers to skills typically acquired after graduation from an entry-level program and requiring considerable training, supervision, and practice to reach competency. Examples of these types of skills include highly technical areas such as those outlined in Table 13.1. Although Table 13.1 provides a sample of such skills, many more exist.

Note that not all high-risk practice areas rely on complex, sophisticated instrumentation. Procedures such as the "blue dye" test for swallowing in patients with tracheotomies, placement of speaking valves, or assessment of complex motor speech disorders require new practitioners to obtain information through multiple sources and to demonstrate satisfactory skill before achieving independence. Failure to do so places patients at health risk and practitioners, as well as institutions, at professional risk.

Acquisition of clinical skill is a career-long process. Speech-language pathologists learn their craft early in their career and modify these skills for its duration. The most challenging aspect of skill acquisition is establishing clinical skills early in the career. During their graduate programs and in their clinical fellowship, speech-language pathologists have the opportunity to receive extensive supervision from experienced supervisors in medical settings. Excellent resources are available to help instructors and supervisors know what content to teach new students and clinical fellows regarding many medical speech-language pathology topics. Available online or by request from ASHA, these practice documents provide information about the knowledge and competencies required for effective practice within a given area. A comprehensive list of available practice guidelines is beyond the scope of this chapter, but a complete listing is available in the speech-language pathology section of the ASHA website (http://www.asha.org). A brief list of examples of these documents is shown in Table 13.2.

There is an important rationale for using professional resources such as the practice documents mentioned above, to guide clinical education. These guidelines can provide an important roadmap to clinical success as they outline background knowledge needed for practice in a given area, review relevant literature specific to the topic, and identify specific procedures and their component skills. They are developed by expert panels of speech-language pathologists who come to consensus about best practice in a given area. Thus, when clinicians use the most current practice guidelines in daily clinical practice, they use information agreed on and approved by their professional association. This reduces the chance that key components of information will be overlooked or that a given educator's/supervisor's bias or lack of currency will interfere with good patient care.

In most cases, the process of clinical education in medical speech-language pathology includes graduate coursework in basic neuroscience, anatomy, and physiology, voice disorders, acquired neurological disorders, and dysphagia. Most master's students in speech-language pathology complete a practicum experience in one or more clinical medical settings. These might include nursing homes, acute-care hospitals, outpatient programs, rehabilitation programs, or private practices. Following completion of their degree, during the clinical fellowship experience, many new speech-language pathologists choose to enter the medical setting. In this first professional experience specialty skills can develop. Although clinicians may require considerable amounts of supervision early in this experience, the fellowship provides a gateway to professional competence and this investment of time and effort can affect career success.

TABLE 13.2   Brief List of Examples of Various Consensus Documents That Guide Practice in Medical Settings

Dysphagia

American Speech-Language-Hearing Association. (2004). Guidelines for speech-language pathologists performing videofluoroscopic swallowing studies. *ASHA Supplement, 24,* 77–92.

American Speech-Language-Hearing Association. (2001). Roles of speech-language pathologists in swallowing and feeding disorders: Technical report. *ASHA 2002 Desk Reference, 3,* 181–199.

American Speech-Language-Hearing Association. (2000). Clinical indicators for instrumental assessment of dysphagia (guidelines). *ASHA Desk Reference, 3,* 225–233.

Dementia

American Speech-Language-Hearing Association. (1988, March). The roles of speech-language pathologists and audiologists in working with older persons. *ASHA Supplement, 30,* 80–84.

Neonates

American Speech-Language-Hearing Association. (2004). Knowledge and skills needed by speech-language pathologists providing services to infants and families in the NICU environment. *ASHA Supplement, 24,* 159–165.

Voice Disorders

American Speech-Language-Hearing Association. (2004). Vocal tract visualization and imaging: Technical report. *ASHA Supplement, 24,* 140–143.

Tracheoesophogeal Puncture

American Speech-Language-Hearing Association. (2004). Evaluation and treatment for tracheoesophageal puncture and prosthesis: Technical report. *ASHA Supplement, 24,* 135–139.

Collaboration with Neuropsychology

Paul-Brown, D., & Ricker, J. H. (2003). Evaluating and Treating Communication and Cognitive Disorders: Approaches to Referral and Collaboration for Speech-Language Pathology and Clinical Neuropsychology. Technical report. *ASHA Supplement, 23,* 47–57.

Motor Speech Disorders

Practice Guidelines for Dysarthria: Evidence for the effectiveness of management of velopharyngeal function. (2003). Available at http://www.ancds.org/practice.html

---

SUMMARY

Medical speech-language pathology contexts provide a rich opportunity for clinical practice. In these settings, speech-language pathologists provide services to children and adults experiencing communication or swallowing difficulties as the result of an underlying disease process or developmental condition. In this chapter we examined the specific demands and opportunities of this environment and highlighted resources available to guide practice. Key ideas include the value of educational preparation and supervision, the importance of finely honed oral and written communication skills, essential development of specialized competencies, and the various roles of speech-language pathologists across medical settings.

THOUGHTS FOR EXPLORATION

1. What specific skills and knowledge are needed for practice in various medical settings? Does practice in this setting appeal to you? Why or why not?
2. What are some valuable resources for practice in medical contexts?

3. What are the speech-language pathologist's responsibilities in completing an effective consultation?
4. What are some examples of "risk" when practicing in a medical setting?
5. Why are professional practice documents valuable in guiding clinical education?

REFERENCES

American Speech-Language-Hearing Association. (2004). Guidelines for speech language pathologists performing videofluoroscopic swallowing studies. *ASHA Supplement 24*, 77–92.

Chi Fishman, G., & Sonies, B. (2002). Kinematic strategies for hyoid movement in rapid sequential swallowing. *JSLHR: Journal of Speech, Language, and Hearing Research, 45*(3), 457–68.

George, K. P., Vikingstad, E., & Cao, Y. Brain imaging in neurocommunicative disorders. (1998). In A. Johnson & B. Jacobson (Eds.), *Medical speech-language pathology: A practitioner's guide.* New York: Thieme.

Golper, L. (1998). *Medical speech pathology sourcebook.* San Diego: Singular.

Golper, L. & Brown, J. (2004). *Business matters: A guide for speech-language pathologists.* Rockville, MD: American Speech-Language-Hearing Association.

Johnson, A., & Jacobson, B. (1998). The scope of medical speech-language pathology. In A. Johnson and B. Jacobson (Eds.), *Medical speech-language pathology: A practitioner's guide* (pp. 3-6). New York: Thieme.

Johnson, A., Valachovic, A. M., & George, K. P. (1998). Speech-language pathology practice in acute care settings: A consultative approach. In A. Johnson and B. Jacobson (Eds.), *Medical speech-language pathology: A practitioner's guide* (pp. 96–130). New York: Thieme.

Karnell, M. P. (1989). Synchronized videostroboscopy and electroglottography. *J Voice, 3*, 68-75.

Karnell, M. P., & Langmore, S. (1998). Videoendoscopy in speech and swallowing for the speech-language pathologist. In A. Johnson and B. Jacobson (Eds.), *Medical speech-language pathology: A practitioner's guide.* New York: Thieme.

Lee, T., Pappius, E., & Goldman, L. (1983). Impact of interphysician communication on the effectiveness of medical consultations. *American Journal of Medicine, 74*, 106–112.

Logemann, J. (1998). Dysphagia: Basic assessment and management issues. In A. Johnson and B. Jacobson (Eds.), *Medical speech-language pathology: A practitioner's guide.* New York: Thieme.

Miller, R., and Groher, M. (1990). *Medical speech pathology.* Rockville, MD: Aspen.

Valachovic, A. M., Smith, B., Elisevich, K., Jacobson, G., & Fisk, J. (1998). Language and its management in the surgical epilepsy patient. In A. Johnson and B. Jacobson (Eds.), *Medical speech-language pathology: A practitioner's guide.* New York: Thieme.

CHAPTER **14**

Speech-Language Pathology in Colleges and Universities

Institutions of Higher Education   In this chapter, higher education institutions refers to colleges and universities that offer academic and clinical programs in speech-language pathology. Of particular importance is the expertise needed to teach and supervise within these settings.

INTRODUCTION

The college or university setting is unique in its multiple missions. These include educating and training future professionals to participate in research and practice. Faculty members, too, have multiple roles and responsibilities.

Traditionally, students provide clinical services under the direct supervision of appropriately credentialed speech-language pathologists. They may work in many types of settings, including on-campus clinics or off-campus clinical facilities. Universities and colleges are the primary bridge to the future of the profession and its practice through discovery of new knowledge, research, and participation in molding the education and careers of the next generation of professionals.

Faculty members in departments of communication sciences and disorders typically hold advanced degrees (master's or doctoral) in speech-language pathology, audiology, speech-language-hearing science, or in a related discipline (Council of Academic Programs in Communication Sciences and Disorders [CAPCSD], 2002). They have experienced many aspects of the university setting and gained perspective on primary university faculty roles that are challenging, exciting, demanding, and rewarding. Ideally, community members see this setting as a resource for the most current research supporting knowledge and practice.

FACULTY COMPOSITION

Faculty in departments of communication sciences and disorders (or any of many program/department names) include knowledgeable scientists and educators whose diverse special interests converge to promote discovery of valuable information, research methodologies, and professional preparation of the next generation of practitioners—clinicians, professors, innovators, administrators, and advocates.

Division 10: Issues in Higher Education is a special-interest division within the American Speech-Language-Hearing Association (ASHA). The specific mission of this division is as follows:

Mission Statement

To foster development of ever-expanding knowledge of instruction, learning strategies, and curriculum to provide the underpinnings of education and skills for practice of the profession. To foster collaboration among programs, faculty, research laboratories, and administration so that common concerns are addressed and resolved in the best interests of our academic members.

http://www.asha.org/members/phd-faculty-research/div_10.htm

This ASHA division has specific goals:

- Disseminate state-of-the-art information on curriculum and instructional practices.
- Provide a forum for discussion and exploration of academically related issues.
- Encourage discussions of curricula and training.
- Develop better and more effective ways to provide academic and clinical education.
- Promote a variety of models for delivery of quality educational and clinical services, while meeting the lifelong learning needs of practitioners.
- Provide members with an understanding of challenges that universities face, while giving them information about quality educational programs.
- Encourage academic debate.
- Encourage cross collaboration and information sharing between professional groups, for example, CAPCSD and ASHA.

Among the varied job descriptions applicable to speech-language pathologists in the university setting, two are typically cited as tenure-earning and non-tenure-earning positions with assignments in teaching, research, clinical supervision, and service. For the purposes of this discussion **clinical faculty** members' primary assignment is clinical teaching and supervision of graduate students in the clinical practicum setting; **academic faculty** members' primary assignment is classroom teaching and research. Most often and indeed ideally, the clinical and academic faculty members are mutually involved in exposing students to theory, knowledge, and practice. Effective communication among faculty members in regard to curriculum issues ensures that the student masters practical/clinical application of theoretical information and research data/findings across the program of study within the major.

Members of departments work together to recruit and retain sufficient qualified faculty members to satisfy the requirements established by ASHA's Council on Academic Accreditation in Audiology and Speech-Language Pathology. ASHA's website (http://www.asha.org) lists the university programs that satisfy these rigorous requirements under the title of "CAA Accredited and Candidate Programs: Online Guide to Graduate Programs." Students should recognize the importance of graduating from an accredited program as required to attain the Certificate of Clinical Competence.

Recruiting and selecting new faculty usually reflect a particular need to fill a vacated position or to increase faculty concentration in a particular area. Departmental faculty work together to ensure that students achieve the best possible preparation to pursue a successful career in the field and then work to develop expertise in their preferred settings and specialties. To achieve this takes collaboration between college or university faculty and prospective employers.

Faculty Concerns

It has become increasingly difficult to attract new faculty into university settings. This may be somewhat attributed to pressures to obtain tenure and promotion and, at one time, lower salaries than the private sector. Fortunately, salary issues are being addressed and additional benefits such as travel, retirement packages, and sabbatical leaves offset the negatives for some. It is often even more difficult to recruit and retain minority faculty members in colleges and universities. According to the Council of Academic Programs in Communication Sciences and Disorders, academic programs in this discipline have fewer than 10% of full-time faculty from ethnic minority groups (Petrosino, Lieberman, & McNeil, 1998).

Programs seek minority representation on faculty to support students from ethnically diverse backgrounds. However, many faculty members of color report a general feeling of lack of support and collegiality that leads them to leave the academic setting in favor of other career opportunities (Gurbitosi, 1999). This has also been reported by nonminority faculty members. In addition, faculty of color who wish to conduct research on minority-related topics believe that their research is undervalued by their peers, who seem to judge such research interests as lacking in academic scholarship. Perceptions by colleagues can certainly influence the outcome of tenure decisions, resulting in fewer minority faculty members obtaining tenure (Battle, 1999). For additional concerns regarding multicultural issues in academic and clinical education, see *A Cultural Mosaic* by Stockman, Boult, & Robinson (2004).

The ideals as well as demands of college/university settings promote faculty excellence and expertise. Ideally, this environment fosters and encourages goals for professional development. To pursue these goals, many university faculty members have duties in three areas: teaching (including clinical supervision), research, and service. The assignments vary with the curricular needs of students in the department, the special abilities and interests of the individual faculty member, and the faculty time available for teaching a particular course among other teaching and research obligations. As a result, this is an excellent context in which to develop recognition as an expert.

TEACHING

Different from the clinician role in other settings, the university faculty (whether academic or clinical faculty) has a primary duty to teach the *how, when, where, what, why, and why not* of the discipline to undergraduate and graduate students. Teaching may take many different forms that include traditional classroom lecture, advanced seminars, clinical instruction in practicum, projects, thesis, laboratory experiences, distance education, conferencing, and use of current available technologies. Regardless of the setting, subject, or class design, the joy and rewards of teaching lie in the success of interested students who seek and grasp the essence of the subject, the value of the information, and the rational placement of the concepts taught in the overall scheme of the discipline.

Academic faculty members typically hold a doctorate within the discipline or a related discipline and primarily support departmental efforts through teaching and research. In addition, they mentor students through classroom teaching and research activities such as directed research projects, specialized clinical projects such as efficacy studies, and thesis and dissertation. They also support their students to develop specialized skills through presentations of their own research projects at professional conferences and conventions as well as through professional publications. Through teaching courses and directing research, academic faculty members provide students with the foundation for the knowledge base of normal development and communication disorders across the lifespan. In addition, academia introduces the student to the keen satisfactions derived from involvement in original research and leads the way to the development of expertise in the discipline.

Clinical faculty members hold at least a master's degree in speech-language pathology or the clinical doctorate (Au.D.) in audiology. They bring to the task of supervision ready insight into interpersonal communication to empower student and novice clinicians to assume with assurance the many responsibilities of the professional practitioner. Clinical faculty members further the knowledge of human communication, its acquisition, differences and disorders through clinical research that demonstrates the ability to identify and address previously unasked or unresolved questions.

Clinical instruction is different from traditional classroom instruction. In a mentored-clinical learning environment the faculty member and student share accountability. The teacher must meet the student's educational/mentoring needs while maintaining service quality and efficacy for the client. The university faculty member, as the student's supervisor, must be capable and comfortable with being one step removed from the client and family. That is, the practicum student must become the primary clinician as one of the initial steps of moving from student to professional.

Often, community practitioners near schools with graduate programs in speech-language pathology may receive clinical appointments to the university department in recognition of clinical teaching they provide to students in their specialized work settings. In other situations, clinical faculty members of the university staff off-campus/community clinical settings to which students are assigned for supervised practicum experiences. Each increases opportunities for consultation and collaboration between the "real world" and the university setting.

It is understandable that clinical practitioners who like to work with direct hands-on diagnosis and treatment may not prefer the one-step-removal from the client. Often, an experienced practicing clinician has a great store of ready knowledge to share with students, and yet by personal preference remains a clinical practitioner rather than a clinical or academic teacher.

RESEARCH

As a part of the traditional code of conduct in the higher education setting, academic faculty members are expected to undertake, continue, and succeed in research efforts. An individual faculty member's research interests tend to follow (or lead) his or her thinking about a segment of the discipline of intense interest over time. The professor's application and amalgam of ideas through research often leads to new—anticipated or unexpected—findings that modify theory and practice in the entire field of speech-language pathology or audiology. Through these experiences and through recognition of research rigor and outcomes, individual college and university faculty members achieve the status of expert in their areas of long-term interest. The culmination of these efforts typically results in publication of articles, monographs, chapters, books, and tests. In addition, faculty members are expected to seek external funding to support the research mission of the college or university program.

Research may be carried out in scientifically equipped laboratories (experimental), or in clinical settings (applied) either in on-campus facilities or in community clinical settings. Currently, clinical techniques, clinical supervision, treatment efficacy, and treatment outcomes are essential clinically based research topics that reflect the move toward evidence-based practice. This type of research is frequently conducted as a part of the blending of academic and clinical efforts.

In days of tight budgets, faculty members are encouraged to seek outside funding through federal grants and foundations to support their personal research interests and the research mission of the college or university program. To write a grant proposal with any hopes of funding, the faculty member must both present a viable research plan and understand and comply with the granting agency's guidelines. Once funded, the grantee becomes the grant administrator and is responsible for using the funds according to the specifications in the approved grant proposal. Thus, in addition to the specific specialization in the discipline of speech-language pathology, the grantee exercises business administration skills in conscientious management of the grant project. This includes selection and oversight of project personnel, execution of the grant plan, and expenditure of funds. Institutional oversight of all funded projects mandates compliance with institutional review boards (IRB), fiscal management, funding agency, and university/college rules and governance. The office of research is often directly responsible to the provost, chancellor, or other chief academic officer of the university/college.

While receiving funding for a grant proposal is highly respected and well recognized within higher educational settings, much viable research occurs without special funding by accumulating data generated through direct daily clinical experience. The value of the findings of any research effort is not necessarily proportional to the amount of outside funding generated to carry it out. Each project results in a report or a paper that disseminates its outcomes, or perhaps in other research proposals that address further aspects of the original project. The results of faculty research generally provide the foundation for published articles in professional journals or for presentations of papers at national and international professional conferences. Such activities provide positive evidence of the university faculty member's contribution to the knowledge bank of the discipline. Many universities support presenters' expenses for travel to participate in such activities.

Published research is another means by which individuals become recognized as having expertise within a specific area. This encourages researchers to explore other options and continue to develop on their road to becoming expert.

SERVICE

Service duties of university faculty vary and represent contributions of the faculty member on professional and university committees, boards, governing agencies, and local/state/national organizations. For example, service may be within the academic department as in chairing one or more committees that help stabilize and manage the organization of the department itself. Service may be to the university or college as a whole, as when faculty members serve on research, tenure and promotion, sabbatical or other committees. Other forms of service promote the profession through membership and elected office in state/regional/national professional organizations.

REWARDS

Working within an academic context has many rewards. These rewards provide incentive for individuals to choose this setting and to devote a professional lifetime to related activities.

Professional Recognition

In academia, the creative, curious mind is employed in discovering and formulating principles and addressing guidelines that define the role of the discipline in an ever-changing society and scope of practice. As a result of these endeavors, faculty members are recognized for their contributions on many levels. Examples of this expertise are readily observable in the efforts of faculty members who have mastered the knowledge base to:

1. Address critical communication/swallowing needs that surface with population changes (e.g., swallowing disorders as researched by Logemann, Groher, and others).

2. Incorporate the inclusion of emerging technologies (e.g., tracheoesophageal puncture techniques as researched by Singer, Blom, Panje, and others; or augmentative communication techniques as researched by Vanderheiden, Yoder, and others).

3. Advocate through definition, diagnosis, interpersonal interaction, guidance, challenge, trials, efficacy, and application as seen in the work of Helm-Estabrooks and Hinckley and others in clinical aphasia trials.

4. Disseminate information related to advancements in the knowledge base and clinical practice through presentations and publications.

The clinical-researchers mentioned here as well as many others have identified a need, devised approaches to resolve problems, and created teachable protocols that have established evidence of desirable outcomes. This level of skill development produces recognition of these individuals as true experts in their chosen areas of practice.

Recognition Within the Department

Opportunities for advancement or recognition are available to both clinical faculty and academic faculty. For example, a clinical teacher/supervisor with outstanding clinical skills who presents consistent excellent organizational and problem-solving skills, and who interacts fairly with colleagues, may be selected by peers to fill the office of clinic director. This honor is in fact a tremendous multifaceted job of organizing and managing the diverse and complex interaction of schedules for staff, faculty, students, clients, and their families. In addition, the clinic director must keep the program current with changes in the clinical education requirements for ASHA certification. The clinic director must ensure that the program offers enough clients and types of disorders to provide sufficient and appropriate supervised practica. This entails maintaining harmony within the clinical faculty, cooperative interaction with the classroom faculty, and effective liaison with the community for off-campus placement of graduate students who have demonstrated competency to undertake that assignment.

Tenure-seeking academic faculty members aim to rise through the ranks of professorship. Faculty members begin as tenure-earning assistant professors. Colleagues within the department examine a candidate's efforts in all areas and the value placed on their outcome before voting whether or not he or she will move from assistant professor to associate professor (typically accompanied by tenure to the college or university), and ultimately to the rank of professor. Awarding tenure removes the risk of dismissal from a professorial position except in rare cases of extreme, grievous breach of institutional principles and policies. Each promotion and the criteria for its achievement are prescribed in the university or college and department governance documents and accompanied by a significant increment in salary. Administrators and department faculty monitor readiness for promotion.

Assistant professors should be mentored by more advanced scholars/researchers/teachers so that they are fully aware of their school's expectations for success. If these faculty members are to succeed in climbing the academic ladder they need to know tenure and promotion expectations and requirements. According to Mendel, Mendel, and Battle (2004):

> Careers in academia are both exciting and rewarding, but communicating those facts often fails. The message sent to future academics tends to focus on day-to-day obstacles and challenges rather than on the long-term benefits of that career path. Instead, we need to inform current graduate students and professionals about the advantages of choosing a career path in academia. (p. 1)

Recognition Within Higher Education

Academic faculty frequently include outstanding individuals interested in the organizational aspects of higher education and whose skills qualify them to pursue administrative positions in academic governance. Department chairpersons often are elected or appointed from among existing faculty. Faculty within departments of communication sciences and disorders often earn recognition as exceptionally competent administrators and are sought for placement in broader aspects of college/university administration. For example, an effective department chair may be invited to assume more rigorous administrative duties over a broader scope of the university governance as in the office of the dean of a college, provost, or president of a university. In fact, many deans, provosts, and presidents in institutions of higher education across the country began their academic careers as speech-language pathologists in departments of communication sciences and disorders.

Robert Ringel (2003) provides an entertaining approach to earning an administrative appointment in a presentation made at the Annual Conference of the CAPCSD in Albuquerque, New Mexico. In this novel presentation, entitled, *The Best Way to Earn an Administrative Appointment*, he indicated several things to keep in mind. A few of these are presented below:

- Establish yourself as an exemplary scholar/teacher.
- Be visible and eligible for the position to which you aspire.
- While waiting to be discovered, continue to develop and fine-tune your skills. Take on additional responsibilities and interact with others from outside your profession.
- Remain active in your specialty area even once you have become an administrator.
- Remain thoughtful and considerate of those you meet on your way up, for you may have to continue interacting with them once you are at the top.
- Administrative stars are rarely born overnight and success in finding the job of your life occurs when preparation meets opportunity.

Sabbatical/Professional Development Leave

Another form of recognition traditionally found available for higher education faculty is the sabbatical, or professional leave. These are releases from assigned duties for a designated period of time (a term or a year) with continuing compensation while pursuing a specific proposal approved by the sabbatical committee of the university. Such periods of release from assigned duties enable the faculty member to devote full time to research, travel, writing, completion of a book, or another planned scholarly activity. This may include creating media for teaching, inventing specialized equipment, or designing therapy materials.

Travel

Faculty rewards may include funds for travel to and participation in national or international professional conferences. Funding may come from the department being represented or the college or university research division. The excitement of conference participation includes opportunities to meet other researchers, witness their contributions, and discuss with them problems, questions, and possibilities for future direction.

GROWING DEMAND FOR ACADEMIC FACULTY

Despite the rewards to be realized, many college and university programs face significant shortages of those who seek to work in higher education. This is reflected in the current scarcity of doctoral-level speech-language pathologists who are potential university faculty. The result is an exceedingly small pool of qualified individuals available today from which to fill the positions emptying rapidly with aging and retirement of the current professors.

It has long been recognized that we are facing a critical shortage of Ph.D.-educated faculty in communication sciences and disorders. Our profession is relatively new and did not have many original faculty members at its start. By the 1990s, many of our early teachers and research-scientists were retiring. During the decades between 2000 and 2020, yet a second generation of researchers and faculty members will be retiring, leaving a considerable number of vacancies in the college and university programs across the United States (http://www.asha.org, retrieved February 15, 2005).

Scott and Wilcox (2002) report only 300 U.S. academic programs in communication sciences and disorders, unevenly distributed throughout the country. For example, Florida has three programs, California has one, and Ohio has six. Among these academic programs, only 61 offer a research Ph.D. in the discipline. Scott and Wilcox further report that 13 states are without doctoral programs in communication sciences and disorders.

In recognition of the shortages of doctoral-educated faculty, ASHA and CAPCSD formed the Joint Ad Hoc Committee on the Shortage of Ph.D. Students and Faculty in Communication Sciences and Disorders. The committee's comprehensive study revealed many interesting findings (CAPCSD report, December 2002):

- All types and degree-level programs must have a stake in fostering and promoting research-based doctoral programs.
- Academic pathways into pre-doctoral education should begin early and at the undergraduate level.
- Doctoral programs must develop a critical mass of students to promote a cohort group of students who can support and encourage each other.
- There is a critical need to prepare future faculty in the scholarship of teaching and learning as well as the challenges they will face in the classroom (http:www.capcsd.org).

Scott and Wilcox (2002) reported that, of approximately 300 students who began their doctoral study in communication sciences and disorders, approximately two-thirds were full-time students and 82% were female. Furthermore, of the students who completed their degrees from 1995 to 2001, 61% assumed faculty positions in colleges and universities. *Crisis in the Discipline: A Plan for Reshaping our Future*, the Ad Hoc Committee Report cosponsored by CAPCSD and ASHA (report available at http://www.asha.org), revealed that in 2001, among all doctoral faculty positions in the field, 6% to 7% were unfilled. The current prediction is that this percentage will continue to climb significantly in the next 10 years. This significant finding has a major impact on all aspects of the discipline and its practice as a profession. See Appendix E for a 10-year history of CAPCSD and ASHA's involvement in the doctoral shortage. The following is taken from the ad hoc report (http://www.asha.org, December, 2002) and summarizes the importance of increasing the number of doctoral-educated individuals who will assume teaching and research positions in colleges and universities.

> The impact of the shortage of Ph.D. students and faculty is widespread. The inability to recruit new Ph.D. faculty is already putting some academic programs at risk for closure. This means potentially fewer professionals, which in turn means fewer and/or poorer services for our clients. Fewer Ph.D. faculty means less research in communication sciences and disorders, which in turn means a slowed growth in our understanding of human communication and a longer time to develop and test improvements to our treatment options. Fewer Ph.D. faculty also means fewer opportunities for doctoral study, which in turn means even fewer Ph.D. faculty. This downward spiral in faculty preparation is perhaps the most significant threat to our future, and highlights the fact that it is the number of faculty (both entering and remaining) in the field that is the ultimate measure of the magnitude of the problem. (pp. 4–5)

Funding Doctoral Education

Funding doctoral-level education is a problem for many students who may want to participate in this educational experience. The two primary sources of funding to support students are usually classified as university funding (internal) or extramural (external) funding. Sources for extramural funding may be federal agencies such as Veterans Affairs or the National Institutes of Health. Other external sources may include foundations such as the ASHA foundation (http://www.ashafoundation.org [new window]) or corporations such as the Starkey First Program (http://www.starkeyfirst.com). Other fellowships

TABLE 14.1   Resources Available for Careers in Higher Education

American Association for Higher Education http://www.aahe.org
Provides information to faculty administrators on issues related to higher education.

American Council on Education http://www.acenet.edu
Provides leadership and advocacy representing views of higher education, especially to academic institutions and policymakers.

The Carnegie Foundation for the Advancement of Teaching http://www.carnegiefoundation.org
Focuses on the scholarship of teaching and provides guidance and leadership in educational research, policy, and practice.

The Chronicle of Higher Education http://www.chronicle.com
This is a major news source for faculty and administrators, providing articles and resources on the most important issues in higher education.

Council of Academic Programs in Communication Sciences and Disorders http://www.capcsd.org
Promotes educational standards and research in the discipline.

Council of Graduate Schools http://www.cgsnet.org
Dedicated to the advancement of graduate education and offers Preparing Future Faculty (PFF) program involving 43 doctoral institutions.

The PEW Charitable Trusts http://www.pewtrusts.com
Supports nonprofit activities in higher education and aims to promote policies and practices that improve education.

target special interests such as a student's minority status as seen in McKnight Fellowships for African-American doctoral students. Nunez (2004) reported that funding sources may be identified by reviewing information on the ASHA website (http://www.asha.org) or by contacting individual programs at universities throughout the United States. A listing of masters and doctoral educational programs may be found on the website for CAPCSD (http://www.capcsd.org).

If fellowships or graduate assistantships are not available, students often can acquire funding for doctoral education through student loans. Most colleges and universities have funding information in their student financial aid office. Another choice for students would be to work part time within the academic program. A doctoral student may be hired to provide research assistance through student employment (sometimes called "other personnel services"-OPS) or, if certified by the American Speech-Language-Hearing Association (CCC-SLP), doctoral students may provide part-time clinical supervision or classroom instruction in the academic program. It is important to remember, however, that clinical instruction is time consuming and may impede progress in a doctoral program. Some doctoral students are already employed in professional service. When this is the case, the student may wish to continue working part time and attend school part time as well. This, in the long run, might reduce the amount of debt at the end of the doctoral program.

It is important to weigh those decisions carefully. Many exciting opportunities await students who decide to return to school to complete doctoral education. Many outstanding career opportunities exist in colleges and universities throughout the United States and world. As the profession continues to grow, along with the need for more research-based clinical intervention, exciting opportunities await bright, young, research-minded faculty in higher education programs. (See Table 14.1 for resources.) The educational setting provides outstanding opportunities to develop unique expertise and to share it with other rising young scholars through teaching and research.

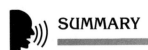 **SUMMARY**

Active participation in the American Speech-Language-Hearing Association through membership in Special Interest Division #10 provides faculty members with outstanding opportunities for continued growth and development of professional skills. Participation in this special interest group also provides members access to state-of-the-art information on teaching, research, and collaboration among programs, faculty, research laboratories, and administration. It furthers development of expertise through shared knowledge. In addition, the Council for Academic Programs in Communication Sciences and Disorders strengthens development of expertise as participants gain a wealth of knowledge concerning issues of the academy, program administration, and current hot topics concerning the profession.

The academic setting allows faculty to develop expertise through research, teaching, and collaboration with knowledgeable colleagues, and to disseminate knowledge to others through published research reports, professional conferences, seminars, and classroom teaching. It is an exciting environment in which to work and one with ever-changing demands and challenges. Career options emerge as one passes through the ranks of the professorate as well as opportunities at all levels of college or university management. Finally, within the discipline of communication sciences and disorders, the projected need for new faculty members across the country means professionals will find ample opportunities for lucrative employment in academic settings for many years to come.

It is, indeed, an exciting, ever-changing environment and one that embraces all aspects of the development of expertise. A career in academia can be satisfying, absorbing, and rewarding.

THOUGHTS FOR EXPLORATION

1. What current trends threaten graduate programs of study?
2. Student-clinicians in graduate programs have access to experts in diagnosis and treatment of a variety of communication disorders. What opportunities allow students to take full advantage of these experts?
3. What are some advantages and challenges experienced by students who have access to a large variety of off-campus sites for clinical observation and practica?

REFERENCES

Battle, D. (1999). Retention of minority faculty in higher education. *Issues in Higher Education, Special Interest Division 10, 3*(2), 7–12.

Gurbitosi, A. (1999). *Diversity Digest: Communicating diversity in higher education.* Washington DC: American Association of Colleges and Universities.

http://www.asha.org

http://www.asha.org

http://capcsd.org

http://starkeyfirst.com

Joint Ad Hoc Committee on the Shortage of Ph.D. Students and Faculty in Communication Sciences and Disorders. (December 2002). *Crisis in the Discipline: A Plan for Reshaping our Future.* American Speech-Language-Hearing Association & Council of Academic Programs in Communication Sciences and Disorders. Available at http://www.capcsd.org

Mendel, L. L., Mendel, M. I., & Battle, D. E. (2004, August 3). Climbing the academic ladder. *ASHA Leader,* 1, 6–7, 23.

Nunez, L. (2004, August 3). Funding a Ph.D. education. *ASHA Leader,* 3, 12.

Petrosino, L., Lieberman, R. J., & McNeil, M. R. (1998). *1996–97 National survey of undergraduate and graduate programs.* Washington DC: Council of Graduate Programs in Communication Sciences and Disorders.

Ringel, R. (2003, April 9–12). *The best way to earn an administrative appointment.* Proceedings of the Annual Conference of the Council on Academic Programs in Communication Sciences and Disorders. Albuquerque, New Mexico.

Scott, C., & Wilcox, K. (2002). The Ph.D. in CSD. *ASHA Leader* online. Available at http://www.asha.org

Stockman, I., Boult, J., & Robinson, G. (2004, July 20). Multicultural issues in academic and clinical education: A cultural mosaic. *ASHA Leader,* 6–7, 20.

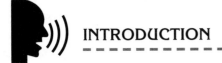

CHAPTER **15**

The First Steps Toward Expertise: Joining the Ranks of the Profession

Clinical Certification and the Clinical Fellowship Year   Achieving the certificate of clinical competence is among the nation's most widely recognized symbol of competency for speech-language pathology and audiology professionals. This is accomplished by completing approved curriculum that meets the highest standards of the professions, earning appropriate clock hours by working with clients across the life span and with a variety of disorders, passing a praxis examination in the area of practice, and completing the Clinical Fellowship Year. (See Chapter 8) The completion of the Speech-Language Pathology Fellowship, is achieved through collaboration between the clinical fellow and a certified mentor. The Clinical Fellow is evaluated across 18 skill statements covering the areas of evaluation, treatment, management, and interaction and includes an assessment of accuracy, consistency, independence, and supervisory guidance. It is only when all requirements have been met that the new professional can begin the journey to developing true expertise.

INTRODUCTION

When that eagerly awaited graduation day has become a fond memory, novice clinicians enjoy a sense of freedom because they are no longer restrained by the need to comply with rules and oversight by school, courses, teachers, and clinical supervisors. However, the newfound realization of success denoted by graduation may also bring recognition that independence carries with it a notable measure of insecurity, uncertainty, and fear. Completion of the master's degree often means that novice clinicians must leave behind immediate familiar support systems such as the safety net provided by clinical supervisors and peers. Although completing academic and clinical requirements has prepared the novice clinician to act independently and competently, early career responsibilities can tax the self-assurance of the best (former) student.

CLINICAL FELLOWSHIP (CF)

Many novice clinicians in speech-language pathology begin their professional career by seeking a clinical fellowship (CF) position in familiar settings where they enjoyed a positive experience during off-campus clinical assignments. Once graduated, the new clinician's first challenge is to cope with all aspects of initiating the next step in career development—finding employment.

TABLE 15.1   A Checklist for Comparing Practice Settings

Considerations	Specific Characteristics

CLINICAL CONCERNS

CLIENT BASE

Client ages: _____Infant _____School Age
_____Toddler _____Adult
_____Preschool _____Geriatric

Diversity of caseload:

_____Articulation _____Hearing
_____Fluency _____Swallowing
_____Voice & Resonance _____Cognitive Aspects of Communication
_____Receptive & Expressive Language
_____Social Aspects of Communication
_____Communication Modalities

Opportunity for specialization Yes_____ No_____
Severity levels _____
Average length of treatment/number of sessions _____

Employees

____Number of SLPs ____Other Disciplines
____Occupational Therapist (OT) ____Support Staff (number and type)
____Physical Therapist (PT)

Referral sources

____Self-referral ____Other SLPs
____Current/previous clients/patients ____Other disciplines
____Hospitals ____Physicians
____Rehabilitation facilities

Physical facility

____Individual offices ____Shared offices
____Appearance (professional, clean, attractive, etc.)

Equipment and materials

____Provided by the facility ____Must purchase

FINANCIAL CONCERNS

Income source

____Salary ____Hourly rate
____Contract ____Percent of revenue

Beginning salary $_____
Timeline for renegotiation _____
Length of contract _____
Noncompete clause Yes_____ No_____
Incentives and rewards

____Sign-on bonus ____Funding for continuing education
____Vacation (length and paid/not paid) ____Flex time
____Payment of professional fees ____Travel reimbursement
____Payment of professional liability insurance

Benefits

____Medical insurance (individual or family) ____Vision insurance
____Dental insurance ____Retirement benefits

PRODUCTIVITY ISSUES

Hrs/week in direct diagnostics/treatment _____
Hrs/week for documentation/billing _____
Other assignments_____ Number of facilities covered_____
Productivity expectations_____%

PROFESSIONAL INVOLVEMENT

____Professional organization involvement
____In-service opportunities
____Opportunities to conduct research
____Opportunities for networking/consultation
____Opportunities for career development
____Opportunities for promotion

COMMUNITY RELATIONS

Reputation of facility Good____ Fair____ Poor____

Community demographics ____Urban ____Rural

____Suburban ____Small town ____Cultural diversity

Features of community ____Potential and established professional networks

____Potential for growth ____Availability of contracts for services

Novice clinicians often look for a CF work setting that satisfies personal preferences for type and severity of communication disorders served, age range of the clientele, physical setting (i.e., hospital, school, private practice, home health, rehabilitation facility), or salary offered. The profession's scope of practice and diversity in practice settings often provide novice clinicians with employment opportunities within commuting distance of home or in distant geographical regions. Some may pursue employment in a local clinic with a reputation for high-quality service well established in the community, while others accept clinical positions in exciting new venues. Each work setting addresses some aspect(s) of the professional scope of practice established for speech-language pathology. The overall need for clinical speech-language pathologists across the United States and the world (as on U.S. military bases, or in schools and clinics in foreign countries) may entice the novice clinician to carefully consider practice setting characteristics and attempt to match those characteristics with personal tastes, preferences, and competencies.

SELECTING THE POSITION THAT IS RIGHT FOR YOU

As we've seen in previous chapters of this book, practice settings tend to be distinctive in a variety of ways. Table 15.1 provides a thorough list of the characteristics and activities you can expect to encounter in typical clinical practice settings that offer speech-language pathology services alone or in conjunction with other health-care and educational services. Novice clinicians can use this list for compiling and comparing information about practice settings. Complete a copy of the checklist for each practice setting you might consider as a possible site for employment. Then, compare the descriptive information and rank them by personal preference. Remember that we do not all share the same personal preferences. It is important to know yourself and what is important to you in an employment setting. This procedure is helpful in eliminating early employment opportunities that compare less favorably with other choices or in deciding between offers of employment from different clinical practice settings.

EMPLOYER EXPECTATIONS

Whatever the position and setting, employment imposes requirements and constraints on each employee. As with other health and human service professions, the speech-language pathologist enters the workplace with credentials that testify to clinical competence. Indeed, it seems that practicing speech-language pathology experts sustain the belief and expectation that well-trained novice clinicians have learned how to learn in a professional clinical environment. The expectation that the novice clinician will continue to increase that type of learning appears to be an unwritten rule applied across settings. Ongoing ready acquisition of new or novel clinical know-how is as critical to an individual's professional success as it is to ensuring the opportunity to achieve clinical expertise.

In the preceding chapters, experts in their areas have given readers a glimpse of how-and-why postgraduate academic and clinical programs are designed to provide graduate students with the basics of the profession. Through academic course work students learn, discuss, and integrate the information. Through supervised practicum each student clinician sharpens personal strengths, minimizes weaknesses, and applies content knowledge to practice of the profession. Through both course work and practicum experience, the novice clinician develops an understanding of the personal and professional value to be gained through incorporating the professional code of ethics into daily practice. The student clinician's personal traits provide the foundation for performance in academic and clinical experiences. As a result, the personal philosophy, preferences, and aspirations of each student clinician are integral to clinical practice. These early experiences set the stage

TABLE 15.2   Views of a Professional Philosophy

Professional Philosophy
By Kellie Coldiron Ellis

I will	**S**peak for those who cannot be heard
I will	**P**rovide for those who need encouragement
I will	**E**mbrace the responsibility of being credentialed
I will	**E**mpower others to achieve their fullest potential
I will	**C**elebrate difference and individuality
I will	**H**old tightly to my goals
I will	**L**earn that fears endanger dreams
I will	**A**cknowledge that independence threatens teamwork
I will	**N**egotiate with others when compromise is needed
I will	**G**uide others and be a leader
I will	**U**nderstand that learning is life long
I will	**A**dvocate for change in policies as needed
I will	**G**overn my actions according to a moral code
I will	**E**mbrace new challenges
I will	**P**ractice professionalism
I will	**A**lways persevere until the challenge is completed
I will	**T**riumph in success
I will	**H**onor the opinions of others
I will	**O**vercome conflict by treating others with respect
I will	**L**earn from mistakes and experiences
I will	**O**pen my heart to the needs of others
I will	**G**row in my respect for my colleagues
I will	**I**nspire my clients to believe in their success
I will	**S**how others ways to achieve success
I will	**T**rust in my abilities

Source: Adapted from Ellis, K. C. (2005, March 1). Professional philosophy. *ASHA Leader,* 39.

for future learning and practice that transition the novice toward becoming more skilled and, finally, an expert.

While a doctoral student at the University of Kentucky, Kellie Coldiron Ellis introduced an interesting approach to developing a professional philosophy. Ellis's *First Person Story* appeared in the *ASHA Leader* (March 1, 2005). In her philosophy, adapted and presented here (Table 15.2), Ellis uses SPEECH LANGUAGE PATHOLOGIST as the beginning letters of statements to reflect her professional philosophy. It is important for novice clinicians to have an understanding of their professional philosophy and how it relates to the mission and ethics of the profession.

The preceding chapters have invited exploration to develop an awareness of **who** the expert clinician is, **what** knowledge and understanding the expert clinician must accumulate; **how** to apply that knowledge to the needs of clients with communication disorders; and **where** the services of the competent-to-expert clinician can be found in modern society. In addition, the chapter content serves as a directory or map that entices and encourages the novice clinician to pursue clinical expertise.

Contributing authors discussed the clinician-as-employee and presented characteristics, tasks, and expectations related to various work settings. They emphasized the experience of the successful clinician in the selected work setting and ways and means to achieve recognition of expertise in each. The information in those chapters helped to identify commonalities among the expectations of the novice and expert clinician.

Employers and clients expect the novice clinician to exhibit the following attributes:

- Demonstrate readiness and willingness to learn about the profession and base evidence of success in academic program and during the CF on personal experiences that may be applied in new contexts.

- Display flexibility and adaptability as demonstrated by their ability to work successfully with numerous supervisors, clients, and peers in the school's clinical practicum program.

- Express a deep and earnest commitment to the function/value of ethical services provided within a given setting.

- Understand that the success of the whole enterprise or institution supports and is supported by the success of the individual professional practitioner.

- Demonstrate expectations and ability to grow and advance in professional matters that meet community needs and expectations.

- Understand the ASHA Code of Ethics and abide by all principles stated therein.

- Self-evaluate and implement plans for professional development.

Likewise, there are expectations about the performance and attributes demonstrated by the expert. The expert clinician applies knowledge acquired from experience to all aspects of service provision and

- Enables the institution/entity (practice setting) to thrive and meet the needs of clients/patients.

- Uses insight into changing community needs and evolving professional demands to enhance clinical services and shape the practice of the profession.

- Is creative and flexible in the approach to each client's diagnosis and treatment.

- Understands and maintains current knowledge of the requirements of federal and state law, policy, and oversight agencies.

- Participates in research to improve efficacy and outcomes for all clients, and to expand the knowledge base of the profession.

- Represents the clinical setting and colleagues in professional and community organizations.

- Stays abreast of current developments in speech-language pathology and learns about new materials, equipment, and techniques.

- Is recognized for exceptional abilities related to the features of expertise (interpersonal skills, professional skills, problem-solving skills, technical skills, knowledge and experience).

FINDING YOUR NICHE

Not all members of the profession, regardless of practice setting, roles, and responsibilities, achieve or sustain all the characteristics that comprise the clinical expert. That is, with the discipline's enormous growth as reflected by the scope of practice, not every clinician is expert in every aspect of the profession. However, successful speech-language pathology professionals must find the specific talents that reflect their individual makeup and pursue their development to the fullest. The melding of all those individual talents makes ours a thriving and continually evolving human services profession.

Whether the graduate or novice clinician is interested in the educational or medical branch of applied speech-language pathology, there is room for the talents and abilities of all within the various practice settings. Few individuals find a single setting that will be a career-long ideal position. The evolving scope of practice, variety of practice settings, and opportunity for retooling allow clinicians to expand their knowledge, skills,

TABLE 15.3 Future Trends and Issues

Future reauthorization of IDEA
Changes to the "No Child Left Behind" program
State legislation affecting provision of services
Changes in Medicaid/Medicare
Role of the speech assistant
New academic degrees (i.e., clinical doctorate)
Growth and expansion of specialty recognition
Methods for conducting clinical education
Recruitment and retention of qualified personnel
Collection and use of efficacy and outcomes data
Growth of specialty recognition
Graying of the professoriate
Critical shortage of clinicians
Aging of the "baby boomers" and the affect on services
Treatment trends
Developments in technology
Expansion of treatment efficacy data bases
Changes in credentialing and accreditation processes
Adequate supervision in pre-professional and clinical fellow positions

and practice across a lifetime in the profession. It is often true that each of us takes a position and molds it as we fit our abilities within the framework of the environment, community, and clientele. Some apply creative talents to a setting and reshape both the environment and the services provided. Such unexpected evolution of services can affect the practice of the profession.

Perhaps one of the most appealing aspects of the discipline of speech-language pathology is its constant change and growth. At local, state, and national professional conferences, discussions include issues of the immediate and distant future. Participation allows members to shape the future of the profession. Professionals must be alert to minute as well as significant changes in professional practice that address special needs of specific clients or a select population. Across a career, as researchers amass more knowledge, practitioners must expand their repertoires. Looking to the future and anticipating societal demands on the discipline, the clinician may study a broad array of interests, issues, and concerns. Table 15.3 lists issues and trends that may affect the education and practice of speech-language pathologists in the future.

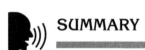 **SUMMARY**

As new ideas become persuasive and accepted, clinicians must often modify procedures and techniques. Some may venture into entirely new areas of diagnosis and treatment. Regular review of research publications is necessary to stay abreast of information. Continuing education opportunities serve practitioners locally and regionally to maintain current knowledge. Often, university faculty and doctoral candidates offer new knowledge, theory, and techniques, as do other members of local, state, and regional professional associations. An example of this is found in the rapid increase in the demand for specialists in swallowing disorders (dysphagia) observed to respond to the well-documented aging of America. Other areas of the practice also have expanded, but perhaps none quite as quickly as the dysphagia practice.

As each practitioner's unique journey toward expertise unfolds, that journey will reveal unpredictable and often unexpected challenges and rewards. The constant, enduring ability to meet those challenges enables the expert clinician to sustain and advance the practice of the profession.

THOUGHTS FOR EXPLORATION

1. How do you think the following issues will affect the profession of speech-language pathology?
   a. The aging of America.
   b. Population mobility—migration, emigration.
   c. The global economy and its effect on the American economy.
2. Complete the checklist in Table 15.1 to describe your "ideal" job in the profession.
3. Design a "futures" list that tells (a) where you expect to be in 10 years, (b) what will be your primary occupation/role and secondary occupation/role at that time, and (c) what will be your relation to the profession of speech-language pathology and all it represents or may come to represent?

REFERENCE

Ellis, K. C. (2005, March 1). Professional philosophy. *ASHA Leader,* 39.

Appendix A
Inventory for Self-Evaluation

Name of Clinician: _____ Date: _____

Setting: _____ Years of Experience: _____

Evaluation Rating Continuum

0 Skill/knowledge is absent or demonstrated inconsistently.

1 Skill/knowledge is developing with input and guidance from supervisor.

2 Skill/knowledge is demonstrated consistently, independently, and intentionally.

3 Skill/knowledge use is intuitive, applied in appropriate situations, applied with a high level of development.

Instructions

Rate your performance or have a supervisor or peer rate your performance on each feature within the Factors of Expertise, using the above rating continuum. Ratings may be completed during direct observation or during observation of a video/audio recorded session. Ratings should include general knowledge of performance within a setting and observed performance.

Skill/knowledge rated as 0 or 1 represents primary targets for improvement. Those rated as 2 should be developed to become intuitive and used at the highest level of performance. Those rated as 3 represent expertise in the associated features.

Analysis of the evaluation data will provide evidence of areas for further development and documentation of progress in professional development when compared to previous evaluations. This information may be used to plan activities for continuing education and professional development.

Features of Interpersonal Skills

_____ Acceptance		_____ Intuition	
_____ Active listening		_____ Nondefensiveness	
_____ Appropriate body language		_____ Open mindedness	
_____ Cooperation		_____ Patience	
_____ Cultural sensitivity		_____ Positive attitude	
_____ Dependability		_____ Reinforcing	
_____ Empathy		_____ Respectfulness	
_____ Enthusiasm		_____ Self-motivation	
_____ Flexibility		_____ Sincerity	
_____ Friendliness		_____ Tactfulness	
_____ Honesty		_____ Tolerance	
_____ Humility		_____ Trustworthiness	

Features of Professional Skills

_____Ability to supervise

_____Awareness of community

_____Compliance with licensure, rules, and regulations

_____Conducting or using relevant research

_____Consultation and collaboration

_____Data collection and dissemination

_____Discharge planning

_____Record keeping

_____Resource management

_____Specialization

_____Utilization of payment methods

Features of Problem-Solving Skills

_____Case management

_____Confidence

_____Decision making

_____Ethical conduct

_____Experience

_____Follow-through

_____Good judgment

_____Making referrals

_____Observant

_____Part-to-whole analysis

_____Professional communication

_____Time management

_____Treatment efficacy

_____Use of task modification techniques

Features of Technical Skills

_____Interpretation of test results and procedures

_____Formulation of appropriate recommendations

_____Selection of appropriate tools and procedures

_____Implementation of diagnostic tools and procedures

_____Oral communication skills

_____Decision making

_____Plan of Care

_____Experience

_____Confidence

_____Ethical conduct

Features of Knowledge and Experience

_____Academic course work

_____Active learner

_____Advanced or specialized knowledge base

_____Continuing education

_____Familiarity with ASHA Code of Ethics

_____Field work experience: internship/externship

_____Knowledge of research methods

_____Lifelong learning

_____Practicum experience

_____Familiarity with Scope of Practice

Summary of Findings:_____

_____

_____

_____

_____

_____

_____

_____

_____

_____

_____

_____

_____

Time Line and Plans for Professional Development:_____

_____

_____

_____

_____

_____

_____

_____

_____

_____

_____

_____

_____

_____

Appendix B
Resources for Evaluating Treatment in Speech-Language Pathology

Agency for Health-Care Research and Quality

American Speech-Language-Hearing Association

American Speech-Language-Hearing Association Desk Reference
http://www.asha.org/members/deskref-journals/deskref/

ASHA Online Journals

ASHA *The Dome*

Academy of Neurological Communication Disorders and Sciences

ANCDS DYSARTHRIA PRACTICE GUIDELINES

Duffy, J. R., & Yorkston, K. M. (2003). Medical interventions for spasmodic dysphonia and some related conditions: A systematic review. *Journal of Medical Speech-Language Pathology, 11*(4).

Duffy, J. R., Yorkston, K. M., Buekelman, D. R., Golper, L. A., Miller, R. M., et al. (2001). *Medical interventions for spasmodic dysphonia and some related conditions: A systematic review* (Tech. Rep. 2). Academy of Neurologic Communication Disorders and Sciences.

Hanson, E. K., Yorkston, K. M., & Buekelman, D. R. (submitted). Speech supplementation techniques for dysarthria: A systematic review. *Journal of Medical Speech-Language Pathology.*

Yorkston, K. M., Hanson, E., & Beukelman, D. (2003). *Speech supplementation techniques for dysarthria: A systematic review* (Tech. Rep. 4). Minneapolis, MN: Academy of Neurologic Communication Disorders and Sciences.

Yorkston, K. M., Spencer, K. A., & Duffy, J. R. (2003). Behavioral management of respiratory/phonatory dysfunction from dysarthria: A systematic review of the evidence. *Journal of Medical Speech-Language Pathology, 11*(2), xiii-xxxviii.

ANCDS COGNITIVE-COMMUNICATIVE PRACTICE GUIDELINES

Kennedy, M., Avery, J., Coelho, C., Sohlberg, M., Turkstra, L., et al. (2002). Evidence-based practice guidelines for cognitive-communication disorders after traumatic brain injury: Initial committee report. *Journal of Medical Speech-Language Pathology, 10*(2), ix-xiii.

Sohlberg, M., Avery, J., Kennedy, M., Coelho, C., Ylvisaker, M., Turkstra, L., et al. (2003). Practice guidelines for direct attention training. *Journal of Medical Speech-Language Pathology, 11*(3), xix-xxxix.

The Cochrane Collection
http://www.cochrane.org
Combined Health Information Database Online
http://www.chid.nih.gov
Clinical Evidence, BMJ Publishing
http://www.clinicalevidence.org
The Communication Disorders Dome
http://www.comdisdome.com
Free Medical Journals
http://www.freemedicaljournals.com
National Institutes on Deafness and Other Communication Disorders
http://www.nidcd.nih.gov

Appendix C
Standards for the Certificate of Clinical Competence in Speech-Language Pathology

Standard I: Degree

Effective January 1, 2005, the applicant for certification must have a master's or doctoral or other recognized post-baccalaureate degree. A minimum of 75 semester credit hours must be completed in a course of study addressing the knowledge and skills pertinent to the field of speech-language pathology.

Implementation

Verification of the graduate degree is required of the applicant before the Certificate is awarded. Degree verification is accomplished by submitting (a) an application signed by the director of the graduate program indicating the degree date, and (b) an official transcript showing that the degree has been awarded. Individuals educated in foreign countries must submit official transcripts and evaluations of their degrees and courses to verify equivalency.

All graduate course work and graduate clinical practicum required in the professional area for which the Certificate is sought must have been initiated and completed at an institution whose program was accredited by the Council on Academic Accreditation in Audiology and Speech-Language Pathology (CAA) of the American Speech-Language-Hearing Association in the area for which the Certificate is sought.

Automatic Approval. If the graduate program of study is completed in a CAA-accredited program and if the program director verifies that all knowledge and skills requirements have been met, approval of the application is automatic, provided that the application for the Certificate of Clinical Competence is received by the National Office in accordance with the time lines stipulated in the chart.

Evaluation Required. The following categories of applicants must submit a completed application for certification, which includes the Knowledge and Skills Acquisition (KASA) summary form for evaluation by the Council for Clinical Certification (CFCC):

a. those who apply after the dates stipulated in the chart

b. those who were graduate students and were continuously enrolled in a CAA-program that had its accreditation withdrawn during the applicant's enrollment

c. those who satisfactorily completed graduate course work, clinical practicum, and knowledge and skills requirements in the area for which certification is sought in a program that held candidacy status for accreditation

d. those who satisfactorily completed graduate course work, clinical practicum, and knowledge and skills requirements in the area for which certification is sought at a CAA-accredited program but (1) received a graduate degree from a program not accredited by CAA; (2) received a graduate degree in a related area; or (3) received a graduate degree from a non-U.S. institution of higher education

The graduate program director must verify satisfactory completion of both undergraduate and graduate academic course work, clinical practicum, and knowledge and skills requirements.

Standard II: Institution of Higher Education

The graduate degree must be granted by a regionally accredited institution of higher education.

Implementation

The institution of higher education must be accredited by one of the following: Commission on Higher Education, Middle States Association of Colleges and Schools; Commission on Institutions of Higher Education, New England Association of Schools and Colleges; Commission on Institutions of Higher Education, North Central Association of Colleges and Schools; Commission on Colleges, Northwest Association Schools and Colleges; Commission on Colleges, Southern Association of Colleges and Schools; and Accrediting Commission for Senior Colleges and Universities, Western Association of Schools and Colleges.

Individuals educated in foreign countries must submit documentation that course work was completed in an institution of higher education that is regionally accredited or recognized by the appropriate regulatory authority for that country. In addition, applicants educated in foreign countries must meet each of the Standards that follow.

Standard III: Program of Study-Knowledge Outcomes

The applicant for certification must complete a program of study (a minimum of 75 semester credit hours overall, including at least 36 at the graduate level) that includes academic course work sufficient in depth and breadth to achieve the specified knowledge outcomes.

Implementation

The program of study must address the knowledge and skills pertinent to the field of speech-language pathology. The applicant must maintain documentation of course work at both undergraduate and graduate levels demonstrating that the requirements in this standard have been met. The minimum 75 semester credit hours may include credit earned for course work, clinical practicum, research, and/or thesis/dissertation. Verification is accomplished by submitting an official transcript showing that the minimum credit hours have been competed.

Standard III-A: The applicant must demonstrate knowledge of the principles of biological sciences, physical sciences, mathematics, and the social/behavioral sciences.

Implementation

The applicant must have transcript credit (which could include course work, advanced placement, CLEP, or examination of equivalency) for each of the following areas: biological sciences, physical sciences, social/behavioral sciences, and mathematics. Appropriate course work may include human anatomy and physiology, neuroanatomy and neurophysiology, genetics, physics, inorganic and organic chemistry, psychology, sociology, anthropology, and nonremedial mathematics. The intent of this standard is to require students to have a broad liberal arts and science background. Courses in biological and physical sciences specifically related to communication sciences and disorders (CSD) may not be applied for certification purposes in this category. In addition to transcript credit, applicants may be required by their graduate program to provide further evidence of meeting this requirement.

Standard III-B: The applicant must demonstrate knowledge of basic human communication and swallowing processes, including their biological, neurological, acoustic, psychological, developmental, and linguistic and cultural bases.

Implementation

This standard emphasizes the basic human communication processes. The applicant must demonstrate the ability to integrate information pertaining to normal and abnormal human development across the life span, including basic communication processes and the impact of cultural and linguistic diversity on communication. Similar knowledge must also be obtained in swallowing processes and new emerging areas of practice. Program documentation may include transcript credit and information obtained by the applicant through clinical experiences, independent studies, and research projects.

Standard III-C: The applicant must demonstrate knowledge of the nature of speech, language, hearing, and communication disorders and differences and swallowing disorders, including the etiologies, characteristics, anatomical/physiological, acoustic, psychological, developmental, and linguistic and cultural correlates. Specific knowledge must be demonstrated in the following areas:

- articulation
- fluency
- voice and resonance, including respiration and phonation
- receptive and expressive language (phonology, morphology, syntax, semantics, and pragmatics) in speaking, listening, reading, writing, and manual modalities
- hearing, including the impact on speech and language
- swallowing (oral, pharyngeal, esophageal, and related functions, including oral function for feeding; orofacial myofunction)
- cognitive aspects of communication (attention, memory, sequencing, problem solving, executive functioning)
- social aspects of communication (including challenging behavior, ineffective social skills, lack of communication opportunities)
- communication modalities (including oral, manual, augmentative, and alternative communication techniques and assistive technologies)

Implementation

The applicant must demonstrate the ability to integrate information delineated in this standard. Program documentation may include transcript credit and information obtained by the applicant through clinical experiences, independent studies, and research projects. It is expected that course work addressing the professional knowledge specified in Standard III-C will occur primarily at the graduate level. The knowledge gained from the graduate program should include an effective balance between traditional parameters of communication (articulation/phonology, voice, fluency, language, and hearing) and additional recognized and emerging areas of practice (e.g., swallowing, upper aerodigestive functions).

Standard III-D: The applicant must possess knowledge of the principles and methods of prevention, assessment, and intervention for people with communication and swallowing disorders, including consideration of anatomical/physiological, psychological, developmental, and linguistic and cultural correlates of the disorders.

Implementation

The applicant must demonstrate the ability to integrate information about prevention, assessment, and intervention over the range of differences and disorders specified in Standard III-C above. Program documentation may include transcript credit and information obtained by the applicant through clinical experiences, independent studies, and research projects.

Standard III-E: The applicant must demonstrate knowledge of standards of ethical conduct.

Implementation

The applicant must demonstrate knowledge of, appreciation for, and ability to interpret the ASHA Code of Ethics. Program documentation may reflect course work, workshop participation, instructional module, clinical experiences, and independent projects.

Standard III-F: The applicant must demonstrate knowledge of processes used in research and the integration of research principles into evidence-based clinical practice.

Implementation

The applicant must demonstrate comprehension of the principles of basic and applied research and research design. In addition the applicant should know how to access sources of research information and have experience relating research to clinical practice. Program documentation could include information obtained through class projects, clinical experiences, independent studies, and research projects.

Standard III-G: The applicant must demonstrate knowledge of contemporary professional issues.

Implementation

The applicant must demonstrate knowledge of professional issues that affect speech-language pathology as a profession. Issues typically include professional practice, academic program accreditation standards, ASHA practice policies and guidelines, and reimbursement procedures. Documentation could include information obtained through clinical experiences, workshops, and independent studies.

Standard III-H: The applicant must demonstrate knowledge about certification, specialty recognition, licensure, and other relevant professional credentials.

Implementation

The applicant must demonstrate knowledge of state and federal regulations and policies related to the practice of speech-language pathology and credentials for professional practice. Documentation could include course modules and instructional workshops.

Standard IV: Program of Study-Skills Outcomes

Standard IV-A: The applicant must complete a curriculum of academic and clinical education that follows an appropriate sequence of learning sufficient to achieve the skills outcomes in Standard IV-G.

Implementation

The applicant's program of study should follow a systematic knowledge- and skill-building sequence in which basic course work and practicum precede, insofar as possible, more advanced course work and practicum.

Standard IV-B: The applicant must possess skill in oral and written or other forms of communication sufficient for entry into professional practice.

Implementation

The applicant must demonstrate communication skills sufficient to achieve effective clinical and professional interaction with clients/patients and relevant others. For oral communication, the applicant must demonstrate speech and language skills in English, which, at a minimum, are consistent with ASHA's most current position statement on students and professionals who speak English with accents and nonstandard dialects. For written communication, the applicant must be able to write and comprehend technical reports, diagnostic and treatment reports, treatment plans, and professional correspondence.

Individuals educated in foreign countries must meet the criteria required by the International Commission of Healthcare Professions (ICHP) in order to meet this standard.

Standard IV-C: The applicant for certification in speech-language pathology must complete a minimum of 400 clock hours of supervised clinical experience in the practice of speech-language pathology. Twenty-five hours must be spent in clinical observation, and 375 hours must be spent in direct client/patient contact.

Implementation

Observation hours generally precede direct contact with clients/patients. However, completion of all 25 observation hours is not a prerequisite to begin direct client/patient contact. The observation and direct client/patient contact hours must be within the scope of practice of speech-language pathology.

For certification purposes, observation experiences must be under the direction of a qualified clinical supervisor who holds current ASHA certification in the appropriate practice area. Such direction may occur simultaneously with the student's observation or may be through review and approval of written reports or summaries submitted by the student. Students may use videotapes of the provision of client services for observation purposes. The applicant must maintain documentation of time spent in supervised observation, verified by the program in accordance with Standards III and IV.

Applicants should be assigned practicum only after they have acquired a sufficient knowledge base to qualify for such experience. Only direct contact with the client or the client's family in assessment, management, and/or counseling can be counted toward practicum. Although several students may observe a clinical session at one time, clinical practicum hours should be assigned only to the student who provides direct services to the client or client's family. Typically, only one student should be working with a given client. In rare circumstances, it is possible for several students working as a team to receive credit for the same session depending on the specific responsibilities each student is assigned. For example, in a diagnostic session, if one student evaluates the client and another interviews the parents, both students may receive credit for the time each spent in providing the service. However, if one student works with the client for 30 minutes and another student works with the client for the next 45 minutes, each student receives credit for the time he/she actually provided services—that is, 30 and 45 minutes, not 75 minutes. The applicant must maintain documentation of time spent in supervised practicum, verified by the program in accordance with Standards III and IV.

Standard IV-D: At least 325 of the 400 clock hours must be completed while the applicant is engaged in graduate study in a program accredited in speech-language pathology by the Council on Academic Accreditation in Audiology and Speech-Language Pathology.

Implementation

A minimum of 325 hours of clinical practicum must be completed at the graduate level. The remaining required hours may have been completed at the undergraduate level at the discretion of the graduate program.

Standard IV-E: Supervision must be provided by individuals who hold the Certificate of Clinical Competence in the appropriate area of practice. The amount of supervision must be appropriate to the student's level of knowledge, experience, and competence. Supervision must be sufficient to ensure the welfare of the client/patient.

Implementation

Direct supervision must be in real time and must never be less than 25% of the student's total contact with each client/patient and must take place periodically throughout the practicum. These are minimum requirements that should be adjusted upward if the student's level of knowledge, experience, and competence warrants. A supervisor must be available to consult as appropriate for the client's/patient's disorder with a student providing clinical services as part of the student's clinical education. Supervision of clinical practicum must include direct observation, guidance, and feedback to permit the student to monitor, evaluate, and improve performance and to develop clinical competence.

All observation and clinical practicum hours used to meet Standard IV-C must be supervised by individuals who hold a current CCC in the professional area in which the observation and practicum hours are being obtained. Only the supervisor who actually observes the student in a clinical session is permitted to verify the credit given to the student for the clinical practicum hours.

Standard IV-F: Supervised practicum must include experience with client/patient populations across the life span and from culturally/linguistically diverse backgrounds. Practicum must include experience with client/patient populations with various types and severities of communication and/or related disorders, differences, and disabilities.

Implementation

The applicant must demonstrate direct client/patient clinical experiences in both diagnosis and treatment with both children and adults from the range of disorders and differences named in Standard III-C.

Standard IV-G: The applicant for certification must complete a program of study that includes supervised clinical experiences sufficient in breadth and depth to achieve the following skills outcomes:

1. Evaluation:
   a. conduct screening and prevention procedures (including prevention activities)
   b. collect case history information and integrate information from clients/patients, family, caregivers, teachers, relevant others, and other professionals

    c. select and administer appropriate evaluation procedures, such as behavioral observations, nonstandardized and standardized tests, and instrumental procedures

    d. adapt evaluation procedures to meet client/patient needs

    e. interpret, integrate, and synthesize all information to develop diagnoses and make appropriate recommendations for intervention

    f. complete administrative and reporting functions necessary to support evaluation

    g. refer clients/patients for appropriate services

2. Intervention:

    a. develop setting-appropriate intervention plans with measurable and achievable goals that meet clients'/patients' needs. Collaborate with clients/patients and relevant others in the planning process

    b. implement intervention plans (involve clients/patients and relevant others in the intervention process

    c. select or develop and use appropriate materials and instrumentation for prevention and intervention

    d. measure and evaluate clients'/patients' performance and progress

    e. modify intervention plans, strategies, materials, or instrumentation as appropriate to meet the needs of clients/patients

    f. complete administrative and reporting functions necessary to support intervention

    g. identify and refer clients/patients for services as appropriate

3. Interaction and Personal Qualities:

    a. communicate effectively, recognizing the needs, values, preferred mode of communication, and cultural/linguistic background of the client/patient, family, caregivers, and relevant others

    b. collaborate with other professionals in case management

    c. provide counseling regarding communication and swallowing disorders to clients/patients, family, caregivers, and relevant others

    d. adhere to the ASHA Code of Ethics and behave professionally

Implementation

The applicant must document the acquisition of the skills referred to in this Standard applicable across the nine major areas listed in Standard III-C. Clinical skills may be developed and demonstrated by means other than direct client/patient contact in clinical practicum experiences, such as academic course work, labs, simulations, examinations, and completion of independent projects. This documentation must be maintained and verified by the program director or official designee.

    For certification purposes, only direct client/patient contact may be applied toward the required minimum of 375 clock hours of supervised clinical experience.

Standard V: Assessment

The applicant for certification must demonstrate successful achievement of the knowledge and skills delineated in Standard III and Standard IV by means of both formative and summative assessment.

    Standard V-A: Formative Assessment   The applicant must meet the education program's requirements for demonstrating satisfactory performance through ongoing formative assessment of knowledge and skills.

Implementation

Formative assessment yields critical information for monitoring an individual's acquisition of knowledge and skills. Therefore, to ensure that the applicant pursues the outcomes stipulated in Standard III and Standard IV in a systematic manner, academic and clinical educators must have assessed developing knowledge and skills throughout the applicant's program of graduate study. Applicants may also be part of the process through self-assessment. Applicants and program faculties should use the ongoing assessment to help the applicant achieve requisite knowledge and skills. Thus, assessments should be followed by implementation of strategies for acquisition of knowledge and skills.

The applicant must adhere to the academic program's formative assessment process and must maintain records verifying ongoing formative assessment. The applicant shall make these records available to the Council for Clinical Certification upon its request. Documentation of formative assessment may take a variety of forms, such as checklists of skills, records of progress in clinical skill development, portfolios, and statements of achievement of academic and practicum course objectives, among others.

Standard V-B: Summative Assessment   The applicant must pass the national examination adopted by ASHA for purposes of certification in speech-language pathology.

Implementation

Summative assessment is a comprehensive examination of learning outcomes at the culmination of professional preparation. Evidence of a passing score on the ASHA-approved national examination in speech-language pathology must be submitted to the National Office by the testing agency administering the examination.

Standard VI: Speech-Language Pathology Clinical Fellowship

After completion of academic course work and practicum (Standard VI), the applicant then must successfully complete a Speech-Language Pathology Clinical Fellowship (SLPCF).

Implementation

The Clinical Fellow may be engaged in clinical service delivery or clinical research that fosters the continued growth and integration of the knowledge, skills, and tasks of clinical practice in speech-language pathology consistent with ASHA's current Scope of Practice. The Clinical Fellow's major responsibilities must be in direct client/patient contact, consultations, record keeping, and administrative duties.

The SLPCF may not be initiated until completion of the graduate course work and graduate clinical practicum required for ASHA certification.

It is the Clinical Fellow's responsibility to identify a mentoring speech-language pathologist (SLP) who holds a current Certificate of Clinical Competence in Speech-Language Pathology. Before beginning the SLPCF and periodically throughout the SLPCF experience, the Clinical Fellow must contact the ASHA National Office to verify the mentoring SLP's current certification status.

Standard VI-A: The mentoring speech-language pathologist and Speech-Language Pathology Clinical Fellow will establish outcomes and performance levels to be achieved during the Speech-Language Pathology Fellowship (SLPCF), based on the Clinical Fellow's academic experiences, setting-specific requirements, and professional interests/goals.

Implementation

The Clinical Fellow and mentoring SLP will determine outcomes and performance levels in a goal-setting conference within 4 weeks of initiating the SLPCF. It is the Clinical Fellow's responsibility to retain documentation of the agreed-upon outcomes and performance levels. The mentoring SLP's guidance should be adequate throughout the SLPCF to achieve the stated outcomes, such that the Clinical Fellow can function independently by the completion of the SLPCF. The Clinical Fellow will submit the SLPCF Report and Rating Form to the Council For Clinical Certification at the conclusion of the SLPCF.

Standard VI-B: The Clinical Fellow and mentoring SLP must engage in periodic assessment of the Clinical Fellow's performance, evaluating the Clinical Fellow's progress toward meeting the established goals and achievement of the clinical skills necessary for independent practice.

Implementation

Assessment of performance may be by both formal and informal means. The Clinical Fellow and mentoring SLP should keep a written record of assessment processes and recommendations. One means of assessment must be the SLPCF Report and Rating Form.

Standard VI-C: The Speech-Language Pathology Clinical Fellowship (SLPCF) will consist of the equivalent of 36 weeks of full-time clinical practice.

Implementation

Full-time clinical practice is defined as a minimum of 35 hours per week in direct patient/client contact, consultations, record keeping, and administrative duties relevant to a bona fide program of clinical work. The length of the SLPCF may be modified for less than full-time employment (FTE) as follows:

15–20 hours/week over 72 weeks
21–26 hours/week over 60 weeks
27–34 hours/week over 48 weeks

Professional experience of less than 15 hours per week does not meet the requirement and may not be counted toward the SLPCF. Similarly, experience of more than 35 hours per week cannot be used to shorten the SLPCF to less than 36 weeks.

Standard VI-D: The Clinical Fellow must submit evidence of successful completion of the Speech-Language Pathology Clinical Fellowship (SLPCF) to the Council for Clinical Certification.

Implementation

The Clinical Fellow must submit the SLPCF Report and Rating Form, which includes the CFSI and documentation of successful achievement of the goals established at the beginning of the SLPCF. This report must be completed by both the Clinical Fellow and the mentoring SLP. The Clinical Fellow must also submit the Employer(s) Verification Form, signed by the employer, which attests to the completion of the 36-week full-time SLPCF or its part-time equivalent.

Standard VII: Maintenance of Certification

Demonstration of continued professional development is mandated for maintenance of the Certificate of Clinical Competence in Speech-Language Pathology. This standard became effective on January 1, 2005. The renewal period will be 3 years. This standard will apply to all Certificate holders, regardless of the date of initial certification.

Implementation

Individuals who hold the Certificate of Clinical Competence (CCC) in Speech-Language Pathology must accumulate 30 contact hours of professional development over the 3-year period in order to meet this standard. At the time of payment of the annual certification fee, individuals holding the CCC in Speech-Language Pathology must acknowledge that they agree to meet this standard. At the conclusion of the renewal period, certified individuals will verify that they have met the requirements of the standard. Individuals will be subject to random review of their professional development activities. If renewal of certification is not accomplished by the end of the 3-year period, certification will lapse. Reapplication for certification will be required, and certification standards in effect at the time of reapplication must be met.

Continued professional development may be demonstrated through one or more of the following options:

- Accumulation of 3 continuing education units (CEUs; 30 contact hours) from continuing education providers approved by the American Speech-Language-Hearing Association (ASHA). ASHA CEUs may be earned through group activities (e.g., workshops, conferences), independent study (e.g., course development, research projects, internships, attendance at educational programs offered by non-ASHA CE providers), and self-study (e.g., videotapes, audiotapes, journals).
- Accumulation of 3 CEUs (30 contact hours) from a provider authorized by the International Association for Continuing Education and Training (IACET).
- Accumulation of 2 semester hours (3 quarter hours) from a college or university that holds regional accreditation or accreditation from an equivalent nationally recognized or governmental accreditation authority.

- Accumulation of 30 contact hours from employer-sponsored in-service or other continuing education activities that contribute to professional development.

Professional development is defined as any activity that relates to the science and contemporary practice of audiology, speech-language pathology, and speech/language/hearing sciences, and results in the acquisition of new knowledge and skills or the enhancement of current knowledge and skills. Professional development activities should be planned in advance and be based on an assessment of knowledge, skills and competencies of the individual and/or an assessment of knowledge, skills, and competencies required for the independent practice of any area of the professions.

For the first renewal cycle, as of January 1, 2005, applications for renewal will be processed on a staggered basis, determined by their initial certification dates. For individuals initially certified before January 1, 1980, professional development activities must be completed between January 1, 2005, and December 31, 2007; for individuals initially certified between January 1, 1980, and December 31, 1989, professional development activities must be completed between January 1, 2006, and December 31, 2008; and for individuals initially certified after January 1, 1990, professional development activities must be completed between January 1, 2007, and December 31, 2009. All individuals will have a 3-year period to complete the process for renewal of certification.

Appendix D
Standards for Accreditation of Graduate Education Programs in Audiology and Speech-Language Pathology

Effective January 1, 1999 (Revised February 2004, May 2004)

Introduction

The American Speech-Language-Hearing Association (ASHA) is committed to ensuring that quality audiology and speech-language pathology services are provided to the public. ASHA believes that the quality of educational preparation for delivery of clinical services is highly correlated with the quality of services provided to the public by certified professional practitioners. Consequently, ASHA maintains a system of accreditation for college and university graduate programs that provide entry-level professional preparation with a major emphasis in audiology and/or speech-language pathology. ("Graduate" refers to post-baccalaureate programs leading to a master's or doctoral degree, including a professional doctoral degree, whether offered through graduate or professional schools.) The accreditation program, which entails both the setting and implementation of standards, is conducted by the Council on Academic Accreditation in Audiology and Speech-Language Pathology (CAA), a council that derives its authority and membership from ASHA but functions autonomously in the accomplishment of its mission and goals. The CAA is recognized by the Council for Higher Education Accreditation and the U.S. Department of Education as the accrediting agency for graduate educational programs that provide entry-level professional preparation with a major emphasis in audiology and/or speech-language pathology.

Underlying the development of these standards is the principle that they should, where possible, be framed in terms of outcome statements. Also included are process standards considered critical to the maintenance of quality educational programs. In recognition and appreciation of the variety of educational goals and missions represented across academic institutions, the standards do not specify a minimum number of faculty required for accreditation. However, the CAA considers a sufficient core of qualified full-time doctoral-level faculty an essential criterion for candidacy, accreditation, and reaccreditation.

Although quality education can be achieved in a variety of ways, the CAA has identified the following five components as essential to quality education in the professions and has established its accreditation standards accordingly.

- Administrative Structure and Governance
- Faculty and Professional Staff
- Curriculum (Academic and Clinical Education)
- Students
- Program Resources

Eligibility

To be eligible for accreditation, programs must meet the following criteria:

1. The applicant institution of higher education within which the speech-language pathology and/or audiology program is housed must hold **regional accreditation** from one of the following six regional accrediting bodies:

- Middle States Association of Colleges and Schools
- New England Association of Schools and Colleges
- North Central Association of Colleges and Schools
- Northwest Association of Schools and Colleges
- Southern Association of Colleges and Schools
- Western Association of Schools and Colleges

For programs in countries outside the United States, the CAA will determine an alternative and equivalent external review process.

2. The institution must offer master's and/or doctoral degree programs that are specifically designed to prepare students for entry into professional practice as audiologists or speech-language pathologists. The applicant institution must apply for accreditation of **all** graduate entry-level preparation programs, whether at the master's or the doctoral level, that it offers in either or both professions (i.e., both master's and doctoral entry-level programs in audiology or both master's and doctoral entry-level programs in speech-language pathology).

3. After December 31, 2003, and until December 31, 2006, the CAA will award Candidacy or initial accreditation only to those graduate education programs in audiology that offer a minimum of 75 graduate semester credit hours that includes (1) academic course work pertinent to the field of audiology, (2) a minimum of 12 months' full-time equivalent supervised clinical practicum, and (3) opportunities for student research consistent with the host university(ies) requirements.

Currently accredited master's programs in audiology continue to be eligible for reaccreditation through December 31, 2006.

After December 31, 2006, the CAA will award **Candidacy, initial accreditation,** or **(re)accreditation** only to doctoral level programs in audiology that offer a minimum of 75 graduate semester credit hours that includes (1) academic course work pertinent to the field of audiology, (2) a minimum of 12 months' full-time equivalent supervised clinical practicum, and (3) opportunities for student research consistent with the host university(ies) requirements. Master's level programs in audiology will no longer be eligible for reaccreditation by the CAA after this date.

(**Note:** The eligibility policy changes described in #3 above were approved November 2003 and May 2004.)

4. The institution must conduct a comprehensive self-analysis that demonstrates how the program meets each of the accreditation standards, and the results of this analysis must be documented in the application for accreditation.

The CAA has adopted the following standards as necessary conditions for accreditation of eligible graduate educational programs. **Programs must satisfy all standards to be awarded accreditation.** The CAA is responsible for evaluating the adequacy of an applicant program's efforts to satisfy each requirement. The CAA recognizes that each of the standards may be satisfied by a variety of means. Compliance with the following standards represents the minimum requirements for accreditation.

Accreditation Standards and Implementation

Standards for accreditation appear in **bold.** Indented information following each standard provides guidance to applicants on how to document compliance and to complete an accreditation application.

Standard 1.0 Administrative Structure and Governance

1.1 The applicant institution of higher education holds regional accreditation.

The applicant institution of higher education within which the speech-language pathology and/or audiology program is housed must hold regional accreditation from one of the following six regional accrediting bodies:

1. Middle States Association of Colleges and Schools,

2. New England Association of Schools and Colleges,

3. North Central Association of Colleges and Schools,

4. Northwest Association of Schools and Colleges,

5. Southern Association of Colleges and Schools,

6. Western Association of Schools and Colleges.

If an applicant program offers academic components that are located outside the region of its home campus and are determined by the regional accrediting body to be separately accreditable, evaluation of the other institution(s) is the responsibility of the region in which it is located. The program should verify to the CAA that all locations in which its academic components are housed are appropriately accredited.

1.2 The program's mission, goals, and objectives are consistent with ASHA-recognized national standards for entry into professional practice and with the mission of the institution.

The application should include the mission statements of the institution and college as well as of the program. The program faculty and professional staff should regularly evaluate the consistency of program and institutional goals and objectives and the extent to which they are achieved. (The implementation statement for Standard 1.2 was revised to ensure programs submit a complete mission statement with the application documentation.)

1.3 The program's faculty/instructional staff have authority and responsibility for making decisions regarding and for conducting the academic and clinical program, including curriculum, within the institution; and the program's faculty/instructional staff have reasonable access to higher levels of administration.

The institution should indicate by its administrative structure that the program's faculty/instructional staff are recognized as a body that can initiate, evaluate, and implement decisions affecting all aspects of the professional education program. Programs without independent departmental status should be particularly clear in describing these aspects of the organizational structure. The program should describe how substantive decisions regarding the academic and clinical programs are initiated, developed, and implemented by the program faculty.

1.4 The individual responsible for the program of professional education seeking accreditation holds a graduate degree with a major emphasis in speech-language pathology, in audiology, or in speech, language, or hearing science, and holds a full-time appointment in the institution. The individual effectively leads and administers the program.

Other areas of major emphasis, such as education of the deaf, special education, reading, administration, speech communication, and otolaryngology, typically do not satisfy this standard. The disciplinary area for a department chair or head is not specified. The individual responsible for the professional program, however, must hold a graduate degree in the profession.

    Effective leadership is provided by the program director with regard to meeting the teaching, research, and service goals of the program and institution.

1.5 Students, staff, and clients are treated equitably—that is, without regard to gender, sexual orientation, age, race, creed, national origin, or disability. The institution and program comply with all applicable laws, regulations, and executive orders pertaining thereto.

The signature of the institution's president or designee affirms the institution's compliance with all applicable federal, state, and local laws, including, but not limited to, the Americans with Disabilities Act of 1990, the Civil Rights Act of 1964, the Equal Pay Act, the Age Discrimination in Employment Act, the Age Discrimination Act of 1975, Title IX of the Education Amendments of 1972 (to the Higher Education Act of 1965), the Rehabilitation Act of 1973, the Vietnam-Era Veterans Readjustment Assistance Act of 1974, and all amendments to the foregoing. The program demonstrates compliance through its policies and procedures.

1.6 The program conducts ongoing and systematic assessment of academic and clinical education and performance of its students and graduates. Students have ongoing opportunity to assess their academic and clinical education program. Results of the assessments are used to plan and implement program improvements that promote high-quality educational experiences for students.

The program should detail the procedures followed in evaluating the quality, currency, and effectiveness of its graduate program, the academic and clinical preparation of its students, the professional performance of its graduates, and the process by which it engages in systematic self-analysis. The plan should indicate the mechanisms used to evaluate each component and the schedule on which the evaluations are conducted. Results of such evaluations should be reported, as well as specific modifications to the program that result from the evaluations. Student performance on the Praxis series examinations in speech-language pathology and/or audiology is an example of an expected outcome measure.

1.7 The program documents student progress toward completion of the graduate degree and professional credentialing requirements and makes this information available to assist students in qualifying for certification and licensure.

The program should maintain accurate and complete records throughout each student's graduate program. It is advisable that forms or computer-tracking programs be developed and used for this purpose. Responsibility for the completion of the records and timetable for completion should be clearly established. Records should be readily available to students upon request. The program should maintain documentation on each student planning to apply for professional credentialing in sufficient detail so that completion of all academic and clinical requirements can be verified.

1.8 The program provides information about the program and the institution to students and to the public that is current, accurate, and readily available.

Catalogs, advertisements, and other publications/electronic media must include accurate information regarding the program's accreditation status, standards and policies regarding recruiting and admission practices, academic offerings, matriculation expectations, graduation rates, academic calendars, grading policies and requirements, and fees and other charges.

Standard 2.0 Faculty/Instructional Staff

2.1 Faculty/instructional staff are qualified and competent by virtue of their education, experience, and professional credentials to provide the academic and clinical education for the program seeking accreditation.

The program should make available vitae of faculty/instructional staff that identify educational background and experience. Qualifications and competence to teach graduate-level courses should be evident in terms of appropriateness of degree level, practical or educational experiences specific to curricular responsibilities in the program, and other indicators of competence to offer graduate education. Individuals providing clinical supervision should hold the appropriate ASHA Certificate of Clinical Competence and other credentials consistent with state requirements. (Implementation statement revised June 25, 1999.)

Doctoral level programs in audiology must demonstrate sufficient doctoral level faculty with appropriate qualifications and expertise to provide the depth and breadth of instruction for the curriculum and must be consistent with the institutional expectations for doctoral programs.

2.2 The number of full-time doctoral-level faculty in speech-language pathology, audiology, and speech, language, and hearing sciences and other full- and part-time faculty/instructional staff is sufficient to meet the teaching, research, and service needs of the program and expectations of the institution.

A sufficient core of qualified full-time speech-language-hearing doctoral-level faculty is essential for accreditation. The program should document that the number of doctoral-level and other faculty/instructional staff is sufficient to offer the curriculum, including its scientific and research components, in such a manner that students can complete the requirements within a reasonable time period. The faculty must have sufficient time for scholarly and creative activities, advising students, participation in faculty governance, and other activities consistent with the institution's expectations. Faculty must be accessible to students. Excessive reliance on ancillary, adjunct, or part-time faculty typically would not meet the standard.

2.3 The institution demonstrates a commitment to the continuity of the program by maintaining a sufficient number of doctoral-level faculty and other instructional staff, with appropriate qualifications to ensure the continued integrity of the program.

Institutional commitment to the program may be demonstrated through documentation of stability of financial support, evidence of recent history of positive actions taken on behalf of the program, long-range academic plans of the institution and program, and promotion/tenure policies for faculty/instructional staff. The program must demonstrate by its allocation of responsibilities that faculty/instructional staff members have the opportunity to meet the institution's criteria for tenure, promotion, or continued employment, in accord with the institution's policies.

2.4 Faculty/instructional staff maintain continuing competence.

The program should describe the mechanism for evaluating the competence of its faculty/instructional staff in academic and clinical teaching, scholarship, and other activities and should provide evidence of the competence of the faculty/instructional staff.

Professional development is one mechanism for supporting continuing competence. The program should demonstrate how support, incentives, and resources are available for the continued professional development of the faculty/instructional staff. Examples of evidence include support for professional travel, release time for professional development, and professional development opportunities on campus.

Standard 3.0 Curriculum (Academic and Clinical Education)

3.1 The curriculum (academic and clinical education) is consistent with the mission and goals of the program and is sufficient to permit students to meet ASHA-recognized national standards for entry into professional practice.

(**Note:** Additional implementation language for Standards 3.1 was added February 2004 and May 2004.)

The program should describe the curriculum leading to a master's or doctoral degree with a major emphasis in speech-language pathology and/or audiology. The program must offer appropriate courses and clinical experiences on a regular basis so that students enrolled in the program may satisfy the requirement for a graduate degree(s) in speech-language pathology and/or audiology for entry into professional practice.

The intent of this standard is to ensure that program graduates are able to meet national standards for entry into professional practice, including ASHA certification. The program may demonstrate how this standard is met by describing outcome evaluations of students' knowledge and skills needed for entry into professional practice.

Master's level programs in audiology must include a minimum of 36 graduate semester credit hours. At least 30 of the 36 semester credit hours of professional course work must be in audiology, including at least 6 hours in hearing disorders and hearing evaluation, at least 6 hours in habilitative/rehabilitative procedures with individuals who have hearing impairment, and at least 6 hours in speech-language pathology. The graduate curriculum must include a minimum of 250 clock hours of supervised clinical observation and supervised clinical practicum in audiology. At least 40 clock hours must be in the area of evaluation of hearing in children, at least 40 clock hours in the evaluation of hearing in adults, at least 80 clock hours in the selection and use of amplification and assistive devices, including a minimum of 10 hours related to children and a minimum of 10 hours related to adults, at least 20 clock hours in the treatment of hearing disorders in children and adults, and at least 20 clock hours in speech-language pathology.

Doctoral level programs in audiology must include a minimum of 75 semester credit hours of post-baccalaureate education culminating in a doctoral degree that is sufficient in depth and breadth for graduates to achieve the knowledge and skills outcomes identified for entry into independent professional practice as identified below. In addition, the curriculum should include appropriate research opportunities, consistent with the specified mission and goals of the program and institutional expectations for doctoral programs.

The doctoral curriculum in audiology also must include a minimum of 12 months' full-time equivalent of supervised clinical practicum during the program of study. The aggregate total of clinical experiences should equal at least 52 weeks. A week of clinical practicum is defined as a minimum of 35 hours per week in direct patient/client contact, consultation, record keeping, and administrative duties relevant to audiology service delivery. Time spent in clinical practicum experiences should occur throughout the graduate program. The program must provide sufficient breadth and depth of opportunities for students to obtain a variety of clinical practicum experiences in different work settings, with different populations, and with appropriate resources and equipment in order to demonstrate skills across the scope of practice in audiology and that are sufficient to enter independent professional practice.

The doctoral academic and clinical curriculum in audiology must include instruction in the areas of (a) foundations of audiology practice, (b) prevention and identification, (c) evaluation, and (d) treatment.

Instruction in foundations of audiology practice should include the following:

- Professional codes of ethics and credentialing
- Patient characteristics (e.g., age, demographics, cultural and linguistic diversity, medical history and status, cognitive status, and physical and sensory abilities) and how they relate to clinical services
- Educational, vocational, and social and psychological effects of hearing impairment and their impact on the development of a treatment program
- Anatomy and physiology, pathophysiology and embryology, and development of the auditory and vestibular systems
- Normal development of speech and language
- Phonologic, morphologic, syntactic, and pragmatic aspects of human communication associated with hearing impairment
- Normal processes of speech and language production and perception over the life span
- Normal aspects of auditory physiology and behavior over the life span
- Principles, methods, and applications of psychoacoustics
- Effects of chemical agents on the auditory and vestibular systems
- Instrumentation and bioelectrical hazards
- Infectious/contagious diseases and universal precautions
- Physical characteristics and measurement of acoustic stimuli
- Physical characteristics and measurement of electric and other nonacoustic stimuli
- Principles and practices of research, including experimental design, statistical methods, and application to clinical populations
- Medical/surgical procedures for treatment of disorders affecting auditory and vestibular systems
- Health care and educational delivery systems
- Ramifications of cultural diversity on professional practice
- Supervisory processes and procedures
- Laws, regulations, policies, and management practices relevant to the profession of audiology
- Manual communication, use of interpreters, and assistive technology

Instruction in prevention and identification of auditory and vestibular disorders should include opportunities for students to, at a minimum, acquire the knowledge and skills necessary to:

- Interact effectively with patients, families, other appropriate individuals, and professionals
- Prevent the onset and minimize the development of communication disorders
- Identify individuals at risk for hearing impairment
- Screen individuals for hearing impairment and disability/handicap using clinically appropriate and culturally sensitive screening measures
- Screen individuals for speech and language impairments and other factors affecting communication function using clinically appropriate and culturally sensitive screening measures
- Administer conservation programs designed to reduce the effects of noise exposure and of agents that are toxic to the auditory and vestibular systems

Instruction in the evaluation of individuals with suspected disorders of auditory, balance, communication, and related systems must include opportunities for students to, at a minimum, acquire the knowledge and skills necessary to:

- Interact effectively with patients, families, other appropriate individuals, and professionals
- Evaluate information from appropriate sources to facilitate assessment planning
- Obtain a case history
- Perform an otoscopic examination
- Determine the need for cerumen removal
- Administer clinically appropriate and culturally sensitive assessment measures
- Perform audiologic assessment using physiologic, psychophysical and self-assessment measures
- Perform electrodiagnostic test procedures
- Perform balance system assessment and determine the need for balance rehabilitation
- Perform aural rehabilitation assessment
- Document evaluation procedures and results
- Interpret results of the evaluation to establish type and severity of disorder
- Generate recommendations and referrals resulting from the evaluation process
- Provide counseling to facilitate understanding of the auditory or balance disorder
- Maintain records in a manner consistent with legal and professional standards
- Communicate results and recommendations orally and in writing to the patient and other appropriate individual(s)
- Use instrumentation according to manufacturer's specifications and recommendations
- Determine whether instrumentation is in calibration according to accepted standards

Instruction in treatment of individuals with auditory, balance, and related communication disorders must include opportunities to, at a minimum, acquire the knowledge and skills necessary to:

- Interact effectively with patients, families, other appropriate individuals, and professionals
- Develop and implement treatment plan using appropriate data
- Discuss prognosis and treatment options with appropriate individuals
- Counsel patients, families, and other appropriate individuals
- Develop culturally sensitive and age-appropriate management strategies
- Collaborate with other service providers in case coordination
- Perform hearing aid, assistive listening device, and sensory aid assessment
- Recommend, dispense, and service prosthetic and assistive devices
- Provide hearing aid, assistive listening device, and sensory aid orientation
- Conduct aural rehabilitation
- Monitor and summarize treatment progress and outcomes
- Assess efficacy of interventions for auditory and balance disorders
- Establish treatment admission and discharge criteria
- Serve as an advocate for patients, families, and other appropriate individuals
- Document treatment procedures and results
- Maintain records in a manner consistent with legal and professional standards
- Communicate results, recommendations, and progress to appropriate individual(s)
- Use instrumentation according to manufacturer's specifications and recommendations
- Determine whether instrumentation is in calibration according to accepted standards

3.2 Academic and clinical education reflects current knowledge, skills, technology, scope of practice, and the diversity of society. The curriculum is regularly reviewed and updated.

The program should provide evidence that the curriculum is regularly and systematically evaluated and updated to reflect current knowledge and scope of practice in the profession(s) and sensitivity to issues of diversity.

3.3 The scientific and research foundations of the professions are evident in the curriculum.

The program should demonstrate how students obtain knowledge in the basic sciences (e.g., biology, physics) and the basic communication sciences (e.g., acoustics, physiological and neurological processes of speech, language, hearing, and linguistics). The curriculum should reflect the scientific bases of the professions and include research methodology, exposure to research literature, and opportunities to participate in research activities.

3.4 The curriculum reflects the interaction and interdependence of speech, language, and hearing in the discipline of human communication sciences and disorders.

The program should demonstrate how students obtain information about the interrelationship of speech, language, and hearing and speech-language pathology and audiology. Programs may detail courses offered, course syllabi, faculty resources, and clinical experiences.

3.5 The academic and clinical curricula reflect an appropriate sequence of learning experiences.

The program should provide evidence of appropriate sequencing of course work and clinical practicum. This should be evident in student records, in examples of typical academic programs, and in the narrative provided within the application.

3.6 The nature, amount, and accessibility of clinical supervision are commensurate with the clinical knowledge and skills of each student.

The program should demonstrate how the nature and amount of supervision are appropriate for the development of clinical skills in individual students.

3.7 The clinical education procedures ensure that the welfare of each client served by students is protected and that the clinical education is in accord with ASHA's Code of Ethics.

The program's written policy statements should describe how this standard is met—in particular, the extent to which students are supervised and have access to needed supervisor consultation when providing services to clients. Procedures for client confidentiality and security of client records should be described.

3.8 Clinical education obtained in external placements is governed by agreements between the program and the external facility and is monitored by program faculty/instructional staff.

The program should provide examples of its written agreements with external facilities and evidence that clinical education in external facilities is monitored by program faculty/instructional staff.

3.9 Academic and clinical education provides students with learning experiences that orient them to providing services in an effective, ethical, legal, and safe manner.

The program should provide evidence (e.g., course syllabi, practicum handbook) that information regarding ethics and legal and safety issues is provided to students. The program should describe how it guides students to assess the effectiveness of their services. The program should also describe how it offers students opportunities to observe and practice in an ethical, legal, and safe manner. Supervisor manuals and lists of student competencies are examples of evidence.

3.10 Clinical education includes a variety of clinical settings, client populations, and age groups.

The program should describe how it ensures that each student is exposed to the varieties described in the standard.

Standard 4.0 Students

4.1 The program criteria for accepting students for graduate study in speech-language pathology and/or audiology are consistent with the institutional policy for admission to graduate study.

A comparison of institutional and program policies should confirm that the program's criteria for admission meet or exceed those of the institution.

4.2 The program makes reasonable adaptations in curriculum, policies, and procedures to accommodate differences among individual students.

The program should provide evidence that its curriculum and its policies and procedures for admission, field placements, and retention of students reflect a respect for and understanding of cultural and individual diversity.

4.3 Students are informed about the program's policies and procedures, degree requirements, requirements for professional credentialing, and ethical practice. A student complaint process is documented.

Programs may provide this information to students through orientation meetings, student handbooks, assigned academic advising, or other means of information dissemination. The program must maintain a record of student complaints and make these available to the CAA upon request. Students should be made aware of the mailing address and telephone number of the CAA in the event they wish to file a complaint.

4.4 Students receive advising on a regular basis that pertains to both academic and clinical performance and progress. Students are also provided information on student support services.

The program should describe how students are advised on a timely and continuing basis regarding their academic and clinical progress. In addition, the program should describe how students receive information about student support services.

Standard 5.0 Program Resources

5.1 The institution provides adequate financial support to the program so that the program can achieve its stated mission, goals, and objectives.

The application should provide evidence that the program receives budgetary allocations for personnel, space, equipment, materials, and supplies appropriate and sufficient for its operation.

5.2 The program has adequate physical facilities (classrooms, offices, clinical space, research laboratories) that are accessible, appropriate, safe, and sufficient to achieve the program's mission, goals, and objectives.

The program should demonstrate that its facilities reflect contemporary standards of ready and reasonable access and use. This includes accommodations for the needs of persons with disabilities consistent with the mandates of the Americans with Disabilities Act of 1990 and the Rehabilitation Act of 1973.

5.3 The program's equipment and educational/clinical materials are appropriate and sufficient to achieve the program's mission, goals, and objectives.

The program should provide evidence that equipment is maintained in good working order and is free of safety hazards. The program must provide evidence of calibration and calibration checks of equipment on a regular schedule. Written records should show that equipment is calibrated to standards specified by the manufacturer, the American National Standards Institute, or other appropriate bodies.

5.4 The program has access to clerical and technical staff, support services, and library and computer resources that are appropriate and sufficient to achieve the program's mission, goals, and objectives.

The program should demonstrate access to appropriate and sufficient resources such as library resources, interlibrary loan services, access to the Internet, and computer laboratory facilities. Support services may be demonstrated by describing how secretarial and technical support are sufficient to assist the program in meeting its mission, goals, and objectives.

5.5 The program has access to a client base sufficiently large and diverse to achieve the program's mission, goals, and objectives and to prepare students to meet the ASHA-recognized national standards for entry into professional practice.

The program should provide information about the size and diversity of the client base and describe the clinical populations available in the practicum facilities where students are placed.

Appendix E
The Doctoral Shortage in CSD:
A Legacy of Concern

Over the past 10 years, ASHA and the Council have invested time and resources in addressing the doctoral shortage. The Joint Ad Hoc Committee on the Critical Shortage of Doctoral Students and Faculty (2001–2001) has reviewed products and publications from these efforts in order to inform its current work.

CAPCSD

- 1983+: Survey of Undergraduate and Graduate Programs
- 1990: Ad Hoc Committee on Doctoral Education (Draft report in 1990 Proceedings)
- 1991: Hixon, T. *Some ingredients of a quality doctoral program in Speech-Language Sciences* (in 1991 Proceedings; see also discussion summary on Hixon's paper); also published in *National Student Speech-Language-Hearing Association Journal, 19,* 89–93 (1991–92)
- 1994: Arranged for a NIDCD Working Group on Research Training Needs of Graduate Programs in Communication Sciences and Disorders, Bethesda, MD: Report from the conference (papers) available on request, CAPCSD
- 1997: Working Group on Doctoral and Postdoctoral Education (http://www.capcsd.org/proceedings/1998/Updates.htm)
- 1998: Wilcox, K. *Replacing the professorate: Perspectives from a doctoral program* (http://www.capcsd.org/proceedings/1998/ReplacingProfessorate.htm)
- 2000: Bernthal, J., & Mendel, M. *Recruiting and retaining doctoral students.* 2000 CAPCSD Proceedings (http://www.capcsd.org/proceedings/2000/00_BernandMend.html)
- 2001: Hurtig, R. *Creative strategies for recruitment of doctoral students: An overview* (http://www.capcsd.org/proceedings/2001/toc2001.html)
- Stathopoulos, E. *Creative strategies for recruiting doctoral students.* The University at Buffalo, SUNY. 2001 CAPCSD Proceedings (http://www.capcsd.org/proceedings/2001/toc2001.html)

ASHA

- 1989: Ad Hoc Committee on Models of Doctoral Education (American Speech-Language-Hearing Association (1991). Report on Doctoral Education. *ASHA, 33* (Suppl. 3), 1–9
- 1994: Research and Scientific Affairs Committee published a Technical Report (American Speech-Language-Hearing Association (1994). The role of research and the state of research training within communication Sciences and disorders. *ASHA, 36*(March), (Suppl. 12), 21–23)
- 1994: Education Future Professionals: Challenges and Solutions for Academia: Blueprint for a New Academic Agenda (American Speech-Language-Hearing Association, 1995)
- 1996: Legislate Council Issues Forum: Scientific Bases of the Discipline and the Professions (presented by Bruce Tomblin, Chair of the Research and Scientific Affairs Committee)
- 1997: Working Group on Recruitment, Retention, and Academic Preparation of Researchers and Teacher-Scholars. (Selected papers, American Speech-Language-Hearing Association, 1997)
- 1997–present: Articles in the *ASHA Leader* by Seymour, Geffner, Logemann, Bernthal, & Creaghead
- 1998: Working Group on Mentoring. Academic Briefing Paper, November 1998
- 1999+: Research in Higher Ed Mentoring Program http://professional.asha.org

- 2000: Survey on the Shortage of Teacher-Scholars
- 2000+: Science and Research Career Forum
- 2000+: Workshops on Grant Writing, Research Integrity, sponsored by Research and Scientific Affairs Committee and ASHA's Science and Research Unit
- 2001: Teleseminar: Doctoral Education in Communication Sciences and Disorders, Schuele & Bacon
- 2002: Doctoral Information Center at ASHA Convention
- 1993 (ASHF and NIDCD): Minghetti, N., Cooper, J., Goldstein, H., Olswang, L., & Warren, S. (1993). *Research mentorship and training in communication sciences and disorders*. Proceedings of a national conference. Rockville, MD: American Speech Language Hearing Foundation
- ASHF: Graduate Scholarships and Research Grants (including the New Investigator Awards)
- 2003: New Century Scholars Program
  - Resources for Funding Doctoral Students: 2002 edition (http://professional.asha.org/resources/grants/funding_students_2001.cfm)
- Lovitts, B., & Nelson, C. (2000). The hidden crisis in graduate education: Attrition from Ph.D. programs. *Academe*, Nov–Dec, 45–50 (http://www.aaup.org/publications/Academe/00nd/ND00LOVI.HTM) (full text)
- The Preparing Future Faculty Program (http://www.preparing-faculty.org/PFFWeb.History.htm)

  ASHA Foundation

Name Index

Adamian, M. S., 44
Allen, F., 90
Alston, R. J., 90
Anderson, J., 32
Anderson, R., 93
Arthur, B., 91
Artiles, A. J., 92, 98

Baker, C., 90
Baker, R. S., 90
Ball, L., 32, 33
Banks, J. A., 90
Barlow, D. H., 69
Barnes, C., 90
Barrera, I., 89, 91
Barrutia, R., 95
Battle, D., 89, 90, 91, 92, 157, 160
Bayles, K., 68
Bazron, B., 89
Bebout, L., 91
Bedore, L., 95
Beeson, P., 68
Bellugi, U., 14
Benjamin, M., 89, 91
Berenson, B., 6
Berliner, D., 32
Besteman, J., 6
Beutler, L. E., 11
Billeaud, U., 15
Birchmeier, A. K., 73
Bland-Stewart, L., 94
Boise, L., 44, 48
Book, C., 50
Boult, J., 157
Bourner, T., 33
Branch, W. T. Jr., 50
Brice, A., 93
Brown, A., 99
Brown, C. P., 90
Brown, J., 143, 144, 145, 149
Brusca-Vega, R., 91

Calderón, J. L., 90
Campbell, L. R., 91, 95
Carhart, Ray, 12
Carkuff, R., 6
Carr, J., 90
Casby, M. W., 111
Castaneda, A., 97
Chabon, S. S., 6, 19, 31, 32
Champion, T., 94, 99
Chang-Rodriguez, E., 95
Chavez, J. A., 91
Cheng, L., 93
Chermak, G. D., 20, 48
Chi, M. T. H., 6, 32
Chinn, P. C., 92
Chomsky, Noam, 12
Clinton, J. J., 6
Cochran-Smith, M., 90
Cohen, J., 67, 92
Cole, L., 10–11
Coleman, T. J., 90
Collier, V., 96

Cornett, B. S., 6, 19, 31, 32
Cox, R. M., 122
Crago, M., 98
Craig, H. K., 94
Cross, T., 89, 93
Crouch, A., 9
Crowell, N. A., 90
Cummins, J., 96

Dalebout, S., 67
Daniels, T., 50
Darrow, M. A., 9
Davis, I. J., 90
Davis, R. N., 72
Davis, T., 90
Dennis, K., 89
DeVellis, B., 44
deVilliers, J., 95
Dollaghan, C., 122
Doody, R. S., 72
Doutis, P., 6
Drew, R. L., 65
Duffy, F. D., 43

Edelstein, R. A., 90
Egan, G., 9
Ehren, B. J., 121
Eicholtz, G. E., 92
Eley, J. W., 50
Ellis, K. C., 168
Elstein, A. S., 27, 32
Emener, W. G., 9, 20, 92
Ericsson, K. A., 6, 32
Ewell, P. T., 81, 83

Farr, M. J., 32
Feltovich, G., 6
Field, T. M., 98
Figueroa, R. A., 96
Fillingham, J. K., 71
Ford, B. A., 95
Forde, T., 99
Fox, J. J., 71
Fradd, S. H., 90
Frago Gracia, J., 95
Frattali, C., 68
Fristoe, M., 94

Galvin, K., 50
Gandara, P., 96
Gansle, K. A., 71
García, S. B., 98
Garrett, Z., 69
Gay, G., 95
Genesee, F., 90, 98
George, K. P., 150
Glasser, R., 6, 32
Goldenberg, C., 98
Goldman, L., 150
Goldman, R., 94
Goldstein, B., 91, 95, 96
Golin, C. E., 44
Golper, L. A., 143, 144, 145, 148, 149
Gonzalez, V., 91

Goodenough, W., 89
Gopaul-McNicol, S., 91, 92
Gould, S. J., 98
Graham, S. J., 32
Graham, S. V., 6, 18, 26, 45, 126
Gray, J. A., 5, 65
Green, L. J., 94
Greenblatt, M., 11
Gresham, F., 70, 71
Grigorenko, E. L., 18
Groher, M., 148
Guerra, P. L., 98
Guilford, A., 12, 14, 18, 45, 126
Gurbitosi, A., 157

Hains, A., 90, 93
Hakuta, K., 95
Hanson, M. J., 91, 92
Harris, J., 98
Harry, B., 92, 94
Haynes, R. B., 5, 65, 66
Heath, S. B., 98
Helfand, M., 111
Hibbard, S., 6, 32
Hidalgo, N. M., 90
Hinckley, J. J., 70, 71
Hodgson, C., 71
Holyoak, K., 32
Homer, A. L., 70
Horvath, J. A., 19
Houser, B., 90
Huffman, N. P., 119

Ingham, J., 70
Isaacs, M., 89, 91
Ivey, Alan, 48, 50

Jackson, R. S., 95
Jacobs, R. L., 6, 32
Jacobson, B., 148, 151
Jacobson, L., 98
Jennings, L., 6, 19
Johnson, A., 148, 150, 151
Johnson, Kenneth O., 59
Johnson, P. R., 142, 143
Johnson, S. M., 71
Johnson, Wendell, 59

Kagan, Norman, 48
Kamhi, A. G., 6, 32, 98
Karlson, E. W., 44
Katz, T., 33
Kayser, H., 91, 96
Kennedy, M., 68
Kierkegaard, S., 6, 13
Kindler, A., 95
Kinlaw, K., 50
Kinnucan-Welsch, K., 121
Kiran, S., 73
Klima, E., 14
Kramer, L., 89, 91
Krampe, R. T., 6, 32
Krashen, S., 93, 95

Subject Index